STRESS LESS LIVE BETTER

For Pregnancy, Postpartum and Early Motherhood

DIANE SANFORD, PhD
AND MEGAN DEMSKY

Praeclarus Press, LLC

www.PraeclarusPress.com

Praeclarus Press, LLC
2504 Sweetgum Lane
Amarillo, Texas 79124 USA
806-367-9950
www.PraeclarusPress.com

DISCLAIMER

The information contained in this publication is advisory only and is not intended to replace sound clinical judgment or individualized patient care. The author disclaims all warranties, whether expressed or implied, including any warranty as the quality, accuracy, safety, or suitability of this information for any particular purpose.

ISBN: 978-1-946665-40-9
©2019 Diane Sanford and Megan Demsky. All rights reserved.

Photography: Kim Wolterman
Cover Design: Ken Tackett
Developmental Editing: Kathleen Kendall-Tackett
Copyediting: Chris Tackett
Layout & Design: Nelly Murariu

CONTENTS

Foreword

I t is a privilege to contribute this Foreword to Diane and Megan's book on the importance of mindfulness for childbearing women and their families. Diane's decades of expertise in the field of perinatal mental health and Megan's first-hand experiences make them perfect co-authors: a master and student team.

Dictionary definitions of mindfulness refer to "a state of being aware." Other related words are wakefulness, attention, alertness, prudence, conscientiousness, consciousness, and observation. Since the 1970s, psychologists and psychiatrists have developed clinical therapeutic practices using mindfulness. Dr. Sanford's application is combined with self-care.

While reading their manuscript, I was reminded of my life journey. I have struggled with mild-to-moderate anxiety and depression my entire life. In childhood and through adolescence, I had daily headaches caused by the stress of school. My pregnancy and postpartum years began in my twenties. Marriage and our experiences with three children and eight grandchildren have been challenging. I had an early onset of menopause. Life has been a roller coaster of emotional upheavals, highs and lows, grief and loss. With some medical intervention, and the occasional counseling session, I have coped. In hindsight, I realize it has been mindfulness and self-care that have brought me joy and good health and kept me emotionally balanced.

Diane has developed five mindfulness-based skillsets that are discussed in this book. They are: Simply Breathe, Soothe Your Body, Savor the Moment, Settle Your Thoughts, and Self-Compassion Always.

These mindfulness exercises reflect what has worked for me. I have used various techniques that help to ease my physical stress, tension, and worry. The first was Transcendental Meditation, known as TM. My husband and I learned to meditate and managed to find time to do so when our children were very young. I remember the sense of peace I felt when chanting my mantra. Our dedication to the practice did not last long. Rather than mediating alone, we began to sit in our Jacuzzi and release our stress in hot water and through conversation. When the children were old enough to be left alone for an hour, we treated ourselves to a date at our local ice cream parlor. We joked and said we were going out for a cup of "soup." It was a fun example of self-care as a couple.

My mother, who lived 91 healthy years, was my role model for regular exercise classes and daily walks. She was in her 80s when she gifted me her black tights. There have been different exercise trends over the years, and I learned yoga decades ago, when it became popular. One of my yoga instructors was a 6-foot, 4-inch man who was also a massage therapist. I decided to invest in weekly massages, and that was over 20 years ago. Now I attend a Pilates class and ice skate. Both require intense concentration and being very much in the moment. I find them to be meditative and calming for my brain, and terrific physical exercise.

Both nutritional intake and sleep hygiene are the foundations of basic life. If only we would practice what our pets teach us: eat well and sleep long. For me, they are paramount. I learned as a child that I loved to sleep and was never a night owl. This was reinforced by my mother saying, "you are doing too much. Take a nap." She also emphasized eating three healthy meals a day. I continue doing as I was taught, and that includes a piece of dark chocolate to end the day.

Breathing is a reflex we take for granted: in and out, repeat. Until I began reflecting on my mindful routines, I had not thought about how well I integrate breath into my life. My flute lessons began in fourth grade, and I started playing the recorder in high school. I cannot remember a time I wasn't singing. Today, I continue these three vigorous breathing activities as a musician. They require concentration, wakefulness, attention, alertness, prudence, conscientiousness, consciousness, and observation. Music keeps me in tune with my body, mind, and soul.

Attaining self-awareness and practicing mindfulness is difficult, especially during life-altering changes, like becoming a mom. It requires daily vigilance, and time to notice and react with positive actions. It is not easy, but it is worth the effort. Join Megan and Diane as they teach you how to stress less and live better on your motherhood journey.

—Jane Honikman, M.S., Founder of
Postpartum Support International

Introduction

For the past 30 years, I've been studying women's health psychology and how women's changing lives, moods, and bodies influence each other. My expertise in perinatal mood and anxiety disorders began when a female psychiatrist, whose office was next door to mine, asked me to see a mom with postpartum depression. I had not given birth to my first child yet but liked working with women and families, so I agreed to see the distressed mom. Eventually, my treatment with her led to a remission of her symptoms. I don't recall what I did, but without realizing it, I had stumbled on to what would become my clinical specialty and a lifelong mission to help women and their families improve their emotional health and well-being.

Before this position, where I was part of a group practice owned by a psychiatrist, I had worked in community mental health seeing children who were referred for behavioral and psychological issues. The children would come for therapy visits once or twice a week, and while they were in my office, things went well. However, when they returned to their homes, many of the negative and disruptive behaviors would resume. As much as I tried to work with their parents, I usually couldn't get them to co-operate with my suggestions. I felt frustrated and sad about their unwillingness to make changes that were in their children's best interest, knowing that their children would suffer from their parents' choices.

Working with pregnant and postpartum patients provided an opportunity to influence families in positive ways from the start. I had focused on child development in my undergraduate studies and knew that depressed and anxious moms were more likely to have children with cognitive, behavioral, social, and emotional problems. Although this is common knowledge now, it wasn't widely understood and accepted then. However, I could see that the moms who recovered from postpartum conditions found that it was much easier to bond with and comfort their babies once they felt better.

Then I had my first child, Jessica. Despite treating postpartum moms and my background in child development, I was miserably unprepared and overwhelmed. Before giving birth, I recall laughing at my OB/GYN when he told me having an infant would be more challenging than getting my PhD or license. How could that be? Like most novice moms, I had no idea of what was ahead. Whether friends share their experiences truthfully or not, you can't imagine before you have a baby how life-altering it is.

My life centered on my daughter, this 7.5 lb wonder who could barely see. In his book, *Happiest Baby on the Block*, pediatrician Harvey Karp says that during the first few months, babies, struggling to transition from their mothers' wombs, are more like fetuses than infants. I agree wholeheartedly. I spent my days tending to her needs, breastfeeding every few hours, changing diapers, wiping spit-up, walking and rocking her, doing her endless laundry, and comforting her.

During my maternity leave, my mom came over daily to provide support physically and emotionally, but instead of taking a nap or resting, I would visit with her or do something around the house, since my husband was still working. LOL. In those days, practicing self-care and making my health and well-being a priority was not on my list. Like many women, my priority was to be a caregiver, not the receiver. I was fortunate that Jessica had a sweet temperament and was easily soothed.

By the end of the first month, I thought things were going reasonably well, only to discover at Jessica's first month's check-up that she wasn't gaining weight. To remedy this, my pediatrician told me I would need to start waking her every few hours, day and night, to breastfeed. The sleep deprivation was torture, and my mood and health tanked. I felt down and that I was failing as a mom. I didn't want to be around my friends, and my usually optimistic outlook dimmed. I spent all my energy breastfeeding and trying to rest in between but my restless mind wouldn't. My OB/GYN scheduled a recheck at 10 weeks because he was concerned that I was starting to have postpartum depression.

Finally, my husband and I decided to start supplementing Jessica with a bottle a couple of weeks before my scheduled return to work. This allowed me to start sleeping again and improving my health and well-being. While I recommended self-care to my clients to recover from their postpartum conditions, I didn't think I needed it myself. Wrong! My postpartum experience convinced me of the importance of self-care for new moms and how critical their health is to their family's well-being.

Going back to work was also good for me. At least there, I felt I was accomplishing something, which helped me regain my confidence and esteem. I suggest that if you have the chance to choose whether to resume work or not, you think about it openly and not make your mind up before your baby is born. I think that you don't know what you may want to do until you become a mom and that this can change over time. Take it one step at a time instead. There is no right or wrong answer about working or staying home, except what's best for you and your family.

When my second daughter Rachel arrived four years later, I diligently practiced self-care. By this time, my dad had retired, and he and my mom would come over daily to help care for the girls and me. My dad would play with my older daughter while my mom and I took turns tending to my younger daughter. I would nap, take showers, and get some time for myself. Most nights, my parents would leave with a warm dinner on the stove. I had no symptoms of depression or anxiety, and thoroughly enjoyed my maternity leave and being with my children. I became convinced that self-care is vital to weathering the storms of new motherhood and for lifelong health and well-being.

After teaching clients for many years, I discovered that while self-care made it possible for them to look at things differently and learn new skills because they were not constantly overwhelmed, it was not enough. Practicing self-care alone would not alleviate the anxiety and worry many of my clients still had. I started investigating other coping skills that would allow them to stress less and enjoy life more. For the past decade, I have focused on mindfulness-based solutions to remedy stress and negative thinking, which is the other skillset in this book.

Mindfulness is a set of strategies that allows you to set aside worries about the future or regrets about the past by directing your attention to the present moment. It has been used for many decades in the United States to improve the health and well-being of people suffering from physical and mental health conditions including anxiety, depression, migraines, heart disease, and irritable bowel syndrome (IBS). More recently, it is being used with pregnancy, childbirth, postpartum, and early parenting, which is what this book is about. I have used it successfully in my own life to deal with personal and health-related challenges, and taught it to hundreds of women going through pregnancy, fertility challenges, and postpartum. Combined with self-care, it can help you weather the changes life brings and enable you to stress less and live better.

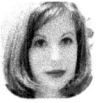

Megan's Mindful-ish Moment: Introduction

Hi, I'm Megan, Diane's coauthor. I am not an expert in women's health, nor have I been practicing mindfulness and meditation for decades. I'm a stay-at-home mom who discovered mindfulness five years ago during my recovery from postpartum depression and anxiety. I know firsthand how well Diane's program works because I was one of the first moms to benefit from it.

Although I have a background in English and writing, I'm not one of those coauthors who's been left to write the whole book while the expert puts her name on the cover. Rather, Diane and I have chosen to team up on this venture to provide our readers with two perspectives: hers, as an experienced psychologist and mindfulness teacher, and mine, as her mindfulness student and parent to a young child. Diane has raised two daughters who have grown into kind, well-adjusted, successful adults, but she will be the first to admit that it has been quite some time since she has been pregnant or parenting an infant or young child. I, on the other hand, am in the parenting trenches right along with you as a mother to a bright, joyful, and, at times, exceedingly stubborn and increasingly sassy 5-year-old. Think of me as your "mom on the street," offering a practical take on the strategies and experiences discussed here.

At times, I think it can be intimidating to learn from people who already seem so skilled, with so many qualifications and letters after their names. I am, like you, a student of mindfulness, and I recognize that I still have much to learn. I am here to share parts of my ongoing journey toward less stress and greater mind-body awareness, from *nama-stay-away-from-me* to *namaste*. I hope I can act as a friend, guiding you through some of the stresses and challenges you'll face learning to stress less and live better. Although we aren't girlfriends in real life, I'd like to think we could be if we knew each other. (I hope you're not too cool for me. I can be kind of a nerd.)

I do not claim to speak for everyone reading this book. I don't know what it's like to be a full-time working mother. Although I spent many years in the workforce and the academic world before having my daughter, I have not (yet) had to juggle full-time employment or education with motherhood as many of you do. I have never experienced being a single mother, either. I have a supportive husband and parents who live nearby, without whose help I could never have found the time to co-write a book. I am sure there are readers out there who have demands on their time that I currently don't, such as caring for an aging parent or working multiple jobs. I recognize that I have been fortunate in many ways.

Once I discovered the benefits of mindfulness and self-care, I couldn't wait to share this discovery with those I cared about. After all, who wouldn't want to reduce their stress? Unfortunately, not everyone is ready to embrace a new mindset. On your journey, you may encounter people who will argue that not everyone has the *luxury* of being able to practice mindfulness and self-care as if emotional stability were comparable to a Caribbean cruise or a pair of Louboutins. (Incidentally, I cannot afford either of these things.) Perhaps there is an optimum way to learn and practice mindfulness, but I'm willing to bet none of us lives at a yoga retreat in the middle of the woods, with endless hours of uninterrupted free time. The good news is that we don't need optimum conditions to reap the benefits of mindfulness practice.

Less stress and a better quality of life are not too much to ask for. We owe it to ourselves to try to achieve this, no matter how busy we are. The question we should be asking ourselves is not whether we have the luxury to practice mindfulness; it's whether we have the luxury *not* to.

About This Book

This book is intended for any woman who is thinking about having a baby, already pregnant, given birth in the past year, or in the throes of parenting toddlers and young children (i.e., early parenting). It is divided into two sections. The first part of the book is about the coping skills you'll need to weather the storm of these significant life changes. Based on Dr. Sanford's experience with hundreds of clients over a 30-year career, specializing in pregnancy, postpartum, motherhood, and emotional health, the Stress Less, Live Better Program for Moms combines self-care practices, with Sanford's Four Pillars of Health and 5 Simple Steps to Stress Less and Live Better.. By learning to calm your mind and body, you can restore your sanity and health, and become an even better mom.

The second half of this book is about learning how to make Dr. Sanford's 5 Simple Steps to Stress Less and Live Better part of your daily life in a way that's practical and NOT overwhelming. As moms, we know that you don't have time when your children are small to sit on a meditation cushion for 45 minutes or stream a 60-minute yoga routine(no one uses VHS tapes, especially not the women of reproductive age who make up our audience)

The great news is that mindfulness is all about taking the moment you're in to calm your body and mind. Many of the exercises in this book take 5 minutes or less, and were designed with moms in mind. Yes, it does require persistent practice and effort to reap the benefits, but this book will teach you how it can be done practically and fit comfortably into your daily life.

So, let's begin.

CHAPTER 1

SELF-CARE ESSENTIALS

Put Your Oxygen Mask on First

Self-care, or convincing moms to take care of themselves, is one of the greatest challenges I face. Most moms put everyone else first if they even put themselves on the list. When I tell them that their health and well-being is equally important as others', they agree and then tell me why that can't be a priority in their lives because they don't have the spare time or energy to expend.

Over the past ten years, it has become popular to say, "Put your oxygen mask on first," which means you can't help someone else if you don't take care of yourself first. Martha Beck, one of this country's best-known life coaches, likes to put it this way: "A conscious parent can help an unconscious child, but a conscious child can't do much to help an unconscious parent." What she means is that we must take good care of ourselves if we want to be able to take good care of others.

Later in this chapter, you can read through the list of why self-care is the last thing most moms think about. As Megan, our "mom on the street," commented earlier about mindfulness, self-care is another aspect of our health we can't afford to neglect. Without self-care, we begin to feel exhausted and overwhelmed. We are irritable and quick to find fault with others, especially our spouses/partners. We have more negative and blaming thoughts. We feel like we are failing miserably and nothing we do is right. These thoughts and feelings are certainly not in the best interest of our babies, our families, and ourselves and not the way to make things better at a time when we are already so stressed and vulnerable.

In the *Tao of Motherhood*, Vimala McClure says, "Taking care of yourself is your right and responsibility. If a mother values herself, her children value her. She teaches self-esteem by her example. Her peaceful demeanor communicates love to all who come in contact with her."

Why Self-Care is Important

In *Life Will Never Be the Same: The Real Mom's Postpartum Survival Guide*, Drs. Dunnewold and Sanford assert that "Practicing self-care is key to a healthy adjustment to motherhood." So, take a deep breath, and repeat out loud; 'My baby needs a mommy, not a martyr!' "Taking care of yourself physically is just as important postpartum as it is when you are pregnant. While pregnant, you devoted lots of energy for doing all you could to ensure a healthy baby. Self-care now is just as essential to being the best mother you can be as was taking vitamins, exercising, and getting regular prenatal care while you were pregnant.

To be a good mother, you must be good to yourself first, both physically and emotionally. This does not mean, of course, that it's okay to neglect your baby's essential needs for food, warmth, cleanliness, or comfort. Babies are very effective when it comes to making sure that their needs are known. Screaming at 4 am, for instance, conveys a pretty clear message; "I need something." What you want to aim for is a balance between your own needs and those of your child. It's best to tackle this issue now because it's one that you'll be facing for the rest of your life.

A pitcher of water provides a clear demonstration of what we mean. Imagine that you are a pitcher of water. You keep pouring out, giving and giving as you take care of the needs of those around you: baby, partner, family, friends. If you do fill the pitcher up again, soon it will be empty. No one is a bottomless pitcher. What do you need to fill up your pitcher again?

The Benefits of Self-Care

When we take good care of ourselves, there are multiple benefits to us as well as others. While self-care may seem self-indulgent, it's not. Self-care enables us to help ourselves and others more.

Self-Care Improves Our Health

Self-care improves our immunity, increases positive thinking, and makes us less susceptible to stress, depression, anxiety, and other emotional health issues. Taking time out to care for ourselves helps remind us and others that our needs are important too. Feeling well-cared for leads to feelings of calm and relaxation and conveys to others that we value ourselves. This can contribute to long-term feelings of well-being.

Self-Care Makes Us Better Caretakers

People who neglect their own needs and forget to nurture themselves are at danger of deeper levels of unhappiness, low self-esteem, and feelings of resentment. Also, sometimes people who spend their time only taking care of others can be at risk of getting burned out on all the giving, which makes it more difficult to care for others or themselves. Taking time to care for yourself regularly can make you a better caretaker for others.

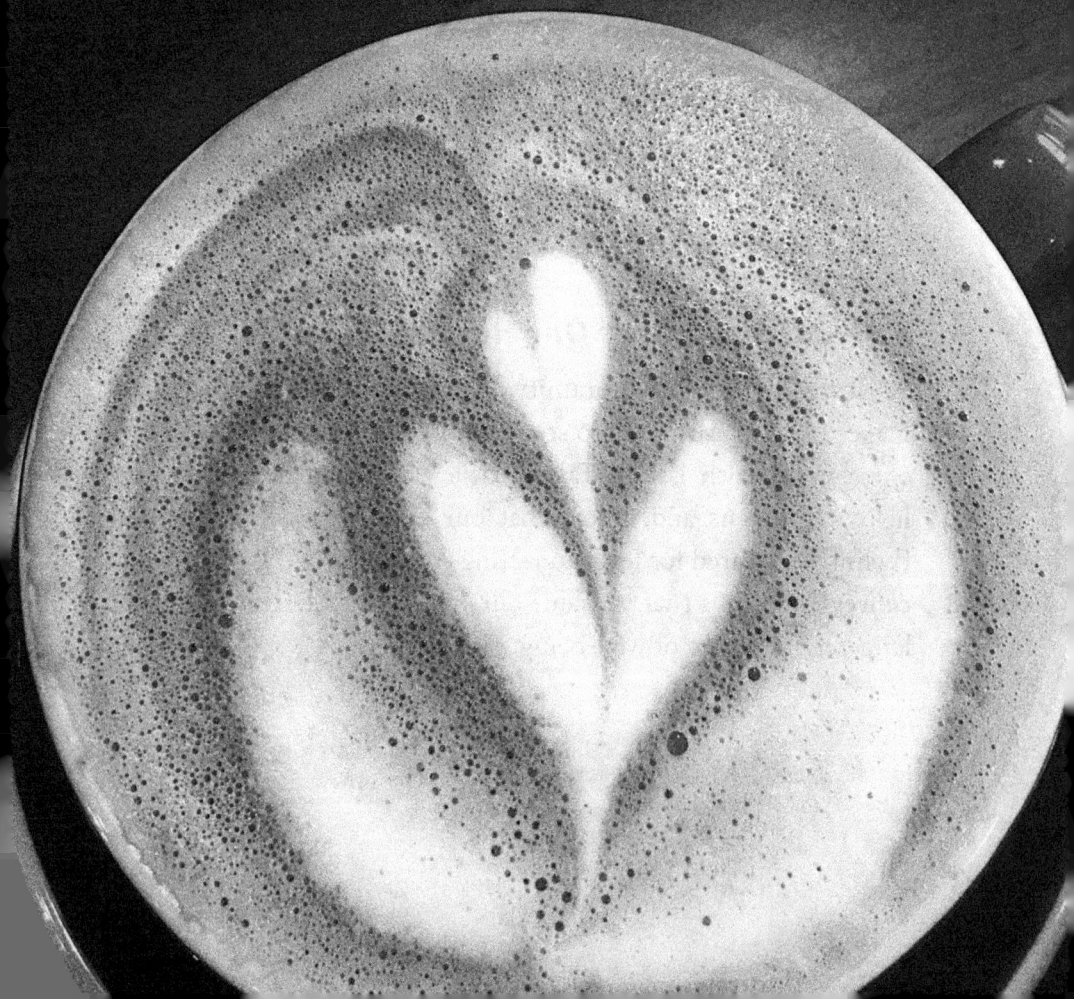

Self-Care Makes Us Better Role Models

By modeling self-care, we are setting a good example for our children. Watching us take time to care for our health and well-being encourages them to do the same, and helps them learn to practice self-care when they are young. Our daughters learn that it is important to put themselves first, at least sometimes, instead of sacrificing their health and well-being to caretaking as many of us were raised to do. It teaches both our sons and daughters self-respect and to be respectful of others because we expect them to value us as we do ourselves.

✏️ *Note-icing Your Experience*

If you like to keep a journal, now would be a good time to get it out and write down your answers to these questions to reflect upon later.

- ❋ How often do you practice self-care? What benefits do you notice?
- ❋ How has practicing self-care helped your health? Made you a better caretaker? Made you a better role model?
- ❋ What did you learn about self-care growing up? Who, if anyone, modeled positive self-care behaviors and how?

Obstacles to Self-Care

One of the most important things you can do to prevent or recover from postpartum emotional problems is to learn to take better care of yourself. As women, this is hard for us to do, even when we aren't facing the physical and emotional demands of infant care, because we never learned to practice self-care. Many of us feel that making our emotional health a priority will interfere with taking good care of our children, partners, families, and friends. The exact opposite is true. The more you care for yourself, the more energy and peace of mind you will have, and the less resentful and stressed you will feel. Take a few minutes now to think about the reasons you do not make your health and well-being a priority and decide what you can do to change this.

Below is a list of common obstacles that prevent women from practicing self-care. Circle those that describe obstacles that get in your way.

* Guilt. Other demands are more important than my own needs.

* My role is to take care of other people. It's what women do.

* Lack of time. I can't find the time to do the things I need to do without adding this.

* I feel selfish when I do something for myself.

* I feel I don't deserve time to do what I want.

* I'm afraid other people won't like me or be mad at me.

* Never learned. My mother never did anything for herself, so why should I?

* Nice girls always put the other person first.

* Perfectionism. It takes all my time to do what needs to be done the "right" way.

* I think I can be healthy without doing this.

✏️ *Note-icing Your Experience*

If you like to keep a journal, now would be a good time to get it out and write down your answers to these questions to reflect upon later.

- ✳ What are some of your most common excuses about why you don't practice self-care?

- ✳ What are some of the reasons from the "Obstacles to Self-Care" list that you don't practice self-care? How did you learn this? Who, if anyone, did you learn it from?

- ✳ What would you say to a friend who wasn't taking good care of herself? What can you tell yourself when you aren't practicing self-care to get started? Keep going?

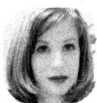

Megan's Mindful-ish Moment: Self-Care

Some people might be resistant to mindfulness and its complementary practices because it all seems too New-Age hippie-dippy-trippy. I am not one of those people. On the hippie continuum, I fall somewhere between liking Birkenstocks and believing in the healing powers of crystals. Meditation, visualization, yoga, Sanskrit mantras, and Buddhist quotes, I'm down for all of that. But when Diane started talking about self-care as a critical component of mindfulness, I balked. "Oh no," I said to myself, "you don't need to remind *me* to practice self-care. I know my weaknesses. I know my tendencies toward laziness and self-centeredness." At the time, although I did practice self-care, I usually saw it as "giving in" to my human frailty, not as a necessary part of emotional and physical well-being. I felt that if I made a point of self-care, instead of continually failing by indulging in it, I would only exacerbate my selfish, negative qualities.

I take full responsibility for laying this guilt trip on myself, but I came by my beliefs honestly. My parents have always been big believers in the Puritan work ethic and pulling yourself up by your bootstraps. Before he retired, my father had had a job since the age of ten, and my mother worked her way through college and lived on four hours of sleep a night for years. Although they had high academic expectations for me, they didn't want me to struggle the way they did, so they happily financed my childhood enrichment activities and didn't expect much from me in the way of household chores. Nevertheless, growing up in this "sleep when you're dead" ideological milieu, I formed the opinion that self-care (I would have called it selfishness) was a luxury and that adulthood was its expiration date.

As it turned out, adulthood in the early aughts tended to be achieved at a different juncture than it did in the early 70s, when my parents came of age. My 20s, often called the "me years," weren't quite the backpacking through Asia, fruit picking at nonprofit organic farms kind of odyssey they were for some of my peers. But I had my share of attempts at finding myself. At 20, I was content to be the center of my universe, but I aspired to the kind of self-discipline and self-sacrifice I thought would be compulsory as a parent. I would have said that I wanted to get all the selfishness out of my system before becoming a mom.

Ten years later, my 30th birthday rolled around, and my husband and I started talking about having children. I felt as ready as anyone ever does to be a parent, except I could still be a little bit selfish and lazy. I still craved "me time," and while I thought I could handle a few sleepless nights, I wasn't prepared for *years* of them. At that time, this felt like weakness. It never occurred to me that the oxygen-mask advice one hears most often while on an airplane was also applicable to the rest of my life.

So yes, I scoffed when Diane suggested I needed to make time for self-care. I would have been a little embarrassed to agree with her right away. *I* didn't need to be reminded about self-care; that was for women with seven kids, three jobs, financial problems, and partners who traveled for business constantly. I was a stay-at-home mom of a newborn, which I thought *should have been* a luxury in and of itself. Then again, the teenage Megan, who had once been constantly distracted by her image in every reflective surface, had become a woman who hadn't looked in a mirror for three days running, not even while brushing her teeth.

You may be thinking, as I did, that the kind of deliberate, restorative, guilt-free self-care Diane recommends is not for you. Perhaps you think you don't have enough time for self-care, or you don't deserve self-care, or both. If you're already a parent, or about to become one, you may feel that the time it takes to take care of yourself would be better spent taking care of your family. You may fear that loving yourself too much will leave too little love to lavish on your precious child.

I am here to tell you that love is not a finite quantity. Love does not follow the laws of thermodynamics. It more closely follows the laws of poetry. Shakespeare wrote,

> *My bounty is as boundless as the sea,*
> *My love as deep; the more I give to thee,*
> *The more I have, for both are infinite. (Romeo and*
> *Juliet, 2.1.175-7)*

Okay, so now we know the sea is not infinite, but love still is. You absolutely can love yourself and love others.

But loving yourself is not just about saying, "I love myself. I'm a smart and capable woman. I'm comfortable in my skin," or similar confidence-boosting affirmations. Loving ourselves is not as much about what we say as it is about what we do. That's where self-care comes in.

Every woman will have her obstacles to self-care. Now that you've read about my reasons to resist self-care, start to examine your own. If you feel you don't need or deserve self-care, where did those feelings come from? Often, the greatest obstacles arise from our worries and fears, not from lack of time. Most of us have at least a little bit of time, even if it's just a few minutes. Conquering our negative feelings and thoughts will take a lot longer than a few minutes, but don't let them prevent you from practicing self-care right away. Once you do, you may find that your mood and energy levels are elevated, and your interactions caring for others are more pleasant and productive.

Even if you've partially accepted the vital role of self-care in your life, you may still want to know what self-care looks like in practice. I wondered that too, because few of the self-care practices I read about or heard from other people resonated with me. They either sounded like humble-brags, like when someone says, "Sure, I take time to relax... by exercising!" or more trouble than they're worth, like taking bubble baths (Aren't those supposed to contribute to urinary tract infections? Plus, I'll have to rinse out the tub afterward). Several years ago, if someone had told me to name two relaxing, restorative things I do purely for myself, I would have said, "Sleep and... um... self-pleasuring?"

While those activities can certainly count as self-care (although I'd prefer you put sleep in a whole other category), so can a host of other things. Some of my (other) self-care practices and rationales behind them include:

✳ Playing Scrabble by myself (uses more brain cells than watching TV, and mood-boosting because I always win).

✳ Reading a good courtroom/forensic/crime thriller (clearly not for work, school, or research purposes).

✳ Getting a manicure. (When you're trying to drag yourself out of bed, you can look at your nails and think, "Hey, I'm 50% ready already!" Good thing I'm not too mathematically accurate early in the morning.)

✳ Trying out new restaurants (tasty, plus no meal planning, food shopping, cooking, or dishes).

✳ Singing karaoke.

✳ Practicing mindful meditation outside on a nice day (relaxing, plus get some Vitamin D).

✳ A glass of wine (to unwind after a harrowing day of parenting) and many others.

Your favorite self-care activities could include crafting, playing pool, dancing, painting, ice fishing, goat yoga – the possibilities are endless. Things I might find stressful, like playing softball or driving, might be excellent stress-relievers for you.

While self-care can take a multiplicity of forms depending on what you find relaxing, there is a caveat. Although I've been researching mindfulness for quite a while, not once have I read anything about the phenomenon of faux self-care.

This can be a real pitfall in our quest for mindfulness, so we should learn to recognize the activities that *seem* like self-care but do not relieve stress the way self-care should. For instance, one woman's self-care may take the form of binge-watching *Real Housewives of the Ninth Circle of Hell*. Afterward, she notices that her irritability has risen and her IQ has dropped. She wonders,

"Isn't self-care supposed to leave me feeling more relaxed and refreshed?" Yes, it is! Our hypothetical woman has succeeded in choosing an activity that she doesn't do for the benefit of someone else. Unfortunately, it doesn't benefit her, either. This doesn't mean that she cannot or should not watch her guilty pleasure, but she can't count it as self-care. (If, on the other hand, mean-girl TV relaxes you and makes you feel like a better version of yourself, watch away!)

While our society seems to have an endless appetite for trashy reality television, watching said programming is also something our society condemns, so it may be easy to determine when we are using it for faux self-care. But what about activities that seem innocuous or even virtuous? When you have been studying and practicing mindfulness for a while, you will hear a lot of people claim that spending time with their children is the greatest, most restorative thing they do for themselves. Besides not having much imagination, I would suggest that these people either a) do not spend nearly as much time with their children as Dave and I spend with ours, b) have the patience of saints (not to mention the similar rapture in martyrdom), or c) are completely clueless. Spending time with your kids has got to be one of the most popular faux-self-care activities in existence. Unless your children are grown (and even sometimes once they are), their needs are going to take precedence over your own, no matter what activity you choose to do together.

Do not mistake what I'm saying here. I don't want anyone to get their knickers in a twist and go Megan-bashing all over the Twittersphere. If you are reading this book, chances are that you're in full-on mom mode, whether you are a parent yet or not. If you already have kids, I know you do, and dare I say, should *enjoy* spending time with your children. If you don't have kids yet, I'm sure you are looking forward to getting to know them. I think Luca is awesome and I love being with her: cuddling with her, playing with her, talking with her, and reading with her. Activities I loved as a child that lost some of their luster as I grew up are now fun again because my child takes joy in them. Of course, being with our kids should be enjoyable and give our lives meaning and all that other great stuff. But self-care it is not.

If parenting feels like self-care to us, perhaps we have lost touch with how it feels to do something purely for ourselves. Parenting is hard work, and we shouldn't have to do it running on empty. There are days when I think, "Luca, I have already pretended to lick the Calico Critters lollipop a hundred times, and if you ask me to do it *one more time*, I am going to lose my mind and my temper!" When a similar scenario arises, if I've been neglecting my self-care, I might voice my frustrations and hurt my child's feelings. When my stress level is lower because I have been diligent with my self-care, I am less quick to become exasperated and, instead, will merely suggest some other play scenario that is a bit less repetitive.

Despite your best efforts at mindfulness and self-care, rest assured that you'll still probably lose it occasionally. I certainly do. For example, one morning I was mentally tallying up all the things I needed to accomplish before and after dropping Luca off at preschool and feeling stressed out and irritable because we were running late. Luca had been pestering me with questions all morning, mostly ones to which she already knew the answer. I set about making my habitual coffee/coconut milk/collagen concoction, Luca "helping" by demanding, "What is that?" about everything I added to the blender. I set the blender on smoothie. I remembered that the day before my husband had said, "You don't have to stand there holding the lid down" and thus felt comfortable enough to walk away for approximately 10 seconds to retrieve coats from the closet. I returned to find that 20 ounces of liquid had exploded all over my kitchen, drenching the cabinets, counters, walls, and floor, not to mention my phone charging station with my phone on it. Luca, standing about 10 feet away, calmly observed, "Mommy, that is a big mess." I then proceeded to let loose a barrage of obscenities the likes of which is seldom heard outside a bar full of drunken sailors. These were directed at the blender, not my child, but I doubt this diminished the overall effect. I finally paused in my venting long enough to draw a few breaths. Luca, being who she is, did not seem particularly upset by the situation or my outburst, but did sum it all up by amending her earlier observation, saying, "Mommy, that is a big F@$!ING mess!"

I didn't receive any incident reports from my daughter's teachers, so I hope she did not repeat any of her new vocabulary words at school. That is not to say she won't someday when one of her classmates drops a tube of loose glitter. In the meantime, I won't be beating myself up too much. Sometimes in life, we will all make big f@$!ing messes, but self-care can help as we try to clean them up.

📄 EXERCISE

Five Minutes for Yourself

You may feel overwhelmed about the barriers to learning this new strategy of self-care. Find a quiet place, and close your eyes. Take three slow, deep breaths. For five minutes, repeat to yourself with each exhaled breath: "Taking care of me benefits my baby." Pick the metaphor that works best for you and picture that image. When you take care of yourself, are you filling your pitcher, building your bank account, or recharging your batteries? Each time thoughts weasel into your head, chastising you that something else is more important than taking time for you, take a deep breath and practice this image and the above phrase. Of course, the baby must come first, but babies are good at making their needs known, and thus met. It's essential to care for yourself to be a good mom.

Remember what Megan, our "mom on the street," said in the introduction. While most of us think we can't afford the luxury of practicing self-care, the truth is that we don't have the luxury of maintaining our health and wellness without it.

CHAPTER 2

THE FOUR PILLARS
OF HEALTH

Women's Changing Lives, Moods, and Bodies

During major life transitions in women's lives, including having a child or going through menopause, many changes occur simultaneously that can create an upheaval in our mind-body health. Let's look at postpartum as an example. Once a woman births her child, and the placenta is delivered, she experiences a hormonal plummet in estrogen and progesterone. This hormonal shift leads to changes in mood and the subsequent mood swings that new moms report. One minute, we feel elated and having a newborn is the best thing ever, and the next, we're filled with dread about being a good mom and how our life has changed.

At the same time, we are sleep deprived, under-nourished, and have little or no time to tend to our own needs. Our sense of identity and self-esteem is disrupted, and we may feel overwhelmed with attempting to meet the competing needs of our baby, our partner, ourselves, and others in our lives. Whether we work inside or outside our homes, there never seems to be enough time in the day to get everything done.

These simultaneous changes create a heightened vulnerability to feeling unsettled and stressed out. Our susceptibility rises to an emotional health condition of postpartum anxiety, depression, or other problems. Current research indicates that 1 in 7 women will have a clinical episode postpartum and it may increase to 1 in 4 in high-risk groups like women with repeated pregnancy loss, complicated pregnancy, or birth trauma.

Learning self-care skills, like the ones discussed in the last chapter, and making certain to apply the Four Pillars of Health talked about in this chapter, can offset some of these unavoidable circumstances. How to combine these with the 5 Simple Steps to Stress Less and Live Better is the subject of the next chapter. While there is no way around the changes that happen during pregnancy and postpartum, many of the moms who work with me find that using these skills helps them to ease stress, anxiety, and worry.

The Journey of Motherhood

Becoming a mom is complicated from the moment you discover you're pregnant, and often even earlier, from the time you begin to imagine having a child. How does this occur? Often before we're pregnant, we tell ourselves stories about what our child may be like, the hopes and dreams we have for them, and what we'll be like as moms. Then when we start experiencing the hormonal, emotional, and situational changes that accompany pregnancy. After having our babies, hormones go haywire, our brains change forever, and life will never be the same. Quite the exhilarating but perilous mind-body rollercoaster ride.

Let's begin by looking more closely at some of the hormone-related changes. During pregnancy, we are flooded with estrogen and progesterone, two main female reproductive hormones that contribute to our brain health and sense of well-being. Estrogen rises rapidly the first few weeks of pregnancy. By week 6, it is three times greater than the highest level it reaches during our monthly cycle. This results in symptoms of irritability, little things bothering us more, being short-fused and unsettled. By second trimester, most women adjust and may feel better than they normally do.

Estrogen is a neurostimulator that helps keep our brains and central nervous system chemistry balanced. As it increases during pregnancy, it may aggravate and cause symptoms of tension and anxiety. Postpartum plummets may result in depression and blue mood. There may also be an intensification of depression and/or anxiety premenstrually once we resume having cycles. Women who are more sensitive to hormonal fluctuations even before becoming pregnant may be more likely to develop anxiety and depression.

Effects of progesterone are significant as well. Progesterone has a calming effect on women's brains, and if it's disrupted, emotional challenges follow. The largest concentration of progesterone receptors is in the limbic area of the brain that is the center of emotion, including anger, rage, and the fight-or-flight response. When it decreases significantly postpartum, women are more likely to experience irritability, negativity, and greater reactivity to stress.

Pregnancy and Postpartum:
The Perfect Storm

If the hormone-related changes we go through aren't enough to disrupt our health and well-being, then the emotional upheaval and situational stressors that come with pregnancy and postpartum can send any woman's life sideways. First comes sleep deprivation, physical exhaustion, depletion of energy, feeding your child every 2-3 hours, and general neglect for one's health.

Then there are the emotional and psychological changes all women experience to some degree. This may result in the first clinical episode of depression and/or anxiety in some women. If this first episode goes un-or-undertreated, some women will relapse or fail to recover fully and be more at risk for subsequent anxiety and depression. One or two in 1000 women will have postpartum psychosis, which is an urgent medical condition in which the life of the mom and baby may be at risk.

Some emotional/psychological stressors include the myth of the perfect mother; feeling you've ruined your life; not being certain you'll ever feel like yourself again; wondering why someone didn't tell you what the reality of caring for an infant was; and feelings of inadequacy, guilt, and shame. Although you're not to blame for feeling like this, you probably will blame yourself and wonder how your baby will ever survive since you're not the perfect mom who is always put together and knows what to do. Honestly, no mom is perfect, but as Dr. Ann Dunnewold says, we can learn to be "good enough."

Here's what motherhood is really like. It is one of life's greatest joys and challenges. It's a constant blend of positive and negative emotions. It is the most important yet most undervalued profession that exists. The hours are long and the return on investment is slow. It is a time of heightened vulnerability and heightened potential, which Piaget called a developmental crisis. It offers the opportunity for growth over time, and enlarging your view of life and yourself in ways you never imagined. The poem that follows below summarizes this.

INSPIRATION
By Patanjali (first to third century, BC)

When you are inspired by some great purpose, some extraordinary project, all your thoughts break their bonds;

Your mind transcends limitations, your consciousness expands in every direction, and you find yourself in a new, great and wonderful world.

Dormant forces, faculties, and talents come alive,

And you discover yourself to be a greater person by far than you ever dreamed yourself to be.

The Four Pillars of Health: Our Bodies and Self-Care

We've already discussed how taking time for self-care is the start of making your health and well-being a priority. The next step is making the four Pillars of Health part of your life. The Four Pillars of Health are nutrition, sleep, exercise, and stress reduction. Be certain that your body is well-nourished and well-rested to supply yourself with the energy needed for exercise and daily living. Taking steps to reduce stress will help keep the other three pillars from becoming disrupted.

1. Nutrition/Nourishment

When you are pregnant or postpartum, it is especially important to eat at regular intervals to keep your body fueled. Substitute more frequent healthy snacks if there isn't time for a full meal. Consume food mindfully for optimal nourishment, both physically and emotionally. Eat without distractions like the TV, cellphones, etc. Eat healthy 75% of the time. Participate in activities that nourish your body and mind.

2. Sleep/Rest

Research shows that adults need 8 to 9 hours of sleep a night to stay sharp mentally and maintain strong immunity. Although this is unlikely postpartum, think about combining sleep and rest for at least 6 hours each day. It is equally important to make time before bed to quiet your mind rather than working until your head hits the pillow. Lack of restful sleep intensifies many physical and emotional health conditions. Rest when you can.

3. Exercise/Movement

Recent studies indicate there are many successful ways to achieve this. Depending on preference, you can exercise 15 to 20 minutes daily, or an hour 3 to 4 times a week. A combination of cardio, strength, and flexibility is best, but any movement is better than none. Again, these are general guidelines, and modifications need to be made postpartum. Remember, periods of activity/energy expenditure require periods of recuperation. Our bodies aren't designed to run full-tilt 24/7. Exercise your mind and relationship muscle too.

4. Stress Reduction

Be aware of physical signs of stress: muscle tension, headaches, and GI symptoms. If these occur, do something restorative–nap, workout, read, journal, or pursue any activity that helps calm your body or mind. Prevent stress from compromising and ultimately ruining your physical and emotional health by doing something. Address warning signs that stress is building and take steps to lessen it. With stress, an ounce of prevention is truly worth a pound of cure.

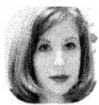

Megan's Mindful-ish Moment: The Four Pillars of Health

The four pillars of health are interconnected. If we neglect one pillar, the three others will suffer as well. If we do nothing to reduce our stress, it can undermine everything else we attempt to do: eat healthfully, exercise, and get a good night's sleep.

Most of us are familiar with the term "stress eating." When I'm neglecting my stress management and lacking in mind-body awareness, I find it difficult to differentiate between feeling unsettled and feeling hungry. One of the many problems with stress eating is how quickly we tend to do it. When we're stressed, we often eat so rapidly that we don't fully enjoy the comfort food we were craving. It takes about 20 minutes for the fullness receptors in our brains to start sending signals to our bodies that we've had enough. You can see why that would be problematic. This is why it is possible to feel ravenous one minute and overstuffed the next.

Unfortunately, we live such fast-paced lives that we often have only 20 minutes—or less—in which to eat. This can make our daily meals seem like stress-related binges. Mindful eating, which involves slowing down and paying attention to what we are consuming, can help us have a more positive relationship with food.

Failing to manage our stress can also affect our exercise habits. Some celebrities and other awesome people exercise to reduce stress. This is a very healthy behavior so, naturally, it is something that rarely occurs to me. Usually, after a stressful day, the last thing I want to do is exercise. What I want is for everyone to leave me alone while I eat half a pizza, down half a bottle of wine, and binge-watch *Game of Thrones*. When my stress is low—either because there is a temporary absence of stressors or, more likely, because I am managing my stress well—I am in a more positive frame of mind. I have more energy and motivation. Then I feel like exercising, as much as I can ever feel like exercising. If you often feel too exhausted and frazzled to exercise, and if you are like me and need to wait until you feel great to get moving, you can keep exercise waiting for a very long time if you don't take steps to reduce your stress.

Speaking of feeling exhausted, when is the last time you consistently got enough sleep? How many times have you found yourself tossing and turning, rehashing the day's events and wishing you had said or done something differently? Have you ever wasted valuable sleep time traveling far back into the past, thinking of witty comebacks to insults you received 20 years ago? Okay, maybe that's just me. At any rate, it is often said that we spend 20% of the time regretting the past and 80% of the time worrying about the future, which leaves us no time to live in the present. This tendency doesn't stop when we go to bed. In fact, in the absence of distractions, our regrets and worries can intensify. Our worries for the future take on larger, often undue significance in the dark. If we lay awake long enough, we begin to worry that we aren't getting enough sleep, wondering how we are going to make it through the next day.

If you want to sleep better, I think Arianna Huffington's book, *The Sleep Revolution*, is a great resource. In it, she quotes psychologist Neil Fiore:

> Calling up the stress response to deal with dangers that are not happening now is like pulling a fire alarm for a fire that happened twenty years ago or to fearing a fire that may happen next year. It would be unfair to the fire department and a misuse of its time and energy to ask firefighters to respond to threats of danger from events that cannot be tackled now.

Similarly, it is a misuse of our time to dwell on the past, which we cannot change, or engage in catastrophic thinking about future events, which we cannot predict or control apart from how we react to them if they do occur. Remember, you are in bed. You are not under any immediate threat; all is well. If you have a to-do list, write it down and then set it aside to deal with in the morning. As we say in mindfulness class, "Breathe in calm, out stress."

✎ *Note-icing Your Experience*

If you like to keep a journal, now is a good time to get it out and write down your answers to these questions to reflect upon later.

* ❋ Which of the above activities are part of your daily routine? Which do you have trouble with?

* ❋ For those that are not part of your daily routine, why not? What would you need to do to make this activity part of your daily routine?

* ❋ What obstacles might you encounter (finding time, feeling guilty, feeling selfish, etc.) that get in your way if you made this activity part of your daily routine? What can you do so that they don't interfere with you taking better care of your health and emotional well-being?

Practice

Choose one of the Four Pillars of Health that aren't currently part of your daily/weekly routine to practice for the next week. Be persistent. Practice daily or several times a week.

When you feel undeserving of the attention and time you take to improve your health and well-being, remind yourself of what Buddha said; "You as much as anyone else in your life are deserving of your love."

Who's Most Likely to Have Pregnancy and Postpartum Anxiety and Depression

Since pregnancy and postpartum are emotionally vulnerable times for women, why do only 1 in 7 (which makes it the most frequent complication of childbirth) experience Postpartum Mood and Anxiety Disorders (PMADs)? I think it's because some women, based on genetics, childhood history, and situational stressors, have more risk of clinical anxiety or depression than others. You've probably heard that heart disease and breast cancer can run in families. So do mood and anxiety conditions, but the difference is that the organ of your body they affect is your brain.

Although many people think that we can "will" our brain to overcome anxiety or depression, this isn't true. Just like someone with diabetes can't "will" their pancreas to produce more insulin, we can't tell our brains to produce more serotonin or dopamine, two of the neurotransmitters that are affected when someone has clinical anxiety or depression. Fortunately for us, health providers and researchers have identified many different risk factors that make some women more likely to have an episode of clinical mood or anxiety symptoms during pregnancy or postpartum than others.

Regarding pregnancy "risk" factor, a summary of 57 studies 1998-2008 indicated that the top three risk factors were life stress, lack of social support, and intimate partner violence. Life stressors ranged from relocating, to loss of a job, to a family member dying. Maternal anxiety, a history of depression, and poor relationship quality emerged as secondary factors. Other factors during pregnancy include a difficult pregnancy; pre-term labor; having multiples; depression and/or anxiety in pregnancy; concerns about your baby's health, especially when there has been bleeding or your baby is measuring small; going through fertility treatments; and prior pregnancy losses or terminations, whatever the circumstances. Women who are sensitive to hormonal fluctuations, or who start having sleep disturbance early in the 3rd trimester, may have more risk too.

In a study of 50 expecting moms, Dr. Ruta Nonacs found that women who were already experiencing symptoms of clinical anxiety and depression in the third trimester had a 94% chance of developing a postpartum clinical condition. This confirmed the importance of women to figure out if they're having a problem with anxiety or depression while they're pregnant, so they can start getting treatment before their baby comes with therapy, medication, or whatever's needed. The sooner moms get help, the sooner they get better.

If you want to explore this more for yourself, then go to Dr. Sanford's website at www.drdianesanford.com, where you can find a quick screen for symptoms of clinical anxiety and depression. If you have a score of 5 or higher on the anxiety or depression scale, tell your health provider right away. If they tell you not to worry, it's normal to feel this way, or don't listen and take you seriously, talk to someone who does and can help you find the care you need. Often, others, like a family member or a close friend who has experienced clinical anxiety or depression can be a good resource in supporting you and helping you find the treatment you need. Many cities have a warmline or mom's line at one of the local hospitals, where trained peer-support volunteers will talk to you and let you know about the resources in your community. Postpartum Support International (PSI), at www.postpartum.net, has a list of all the state peer-support coordinators that participate in their network, as well as therapists who specialize in Perinatal Mood and Anxiety Disorders listed by state with contact information.

Regarding pregnancy AND postpartum, the following factors seem to put a woman at greater risk for either. These include a personal history of anxiety, depression, OCD, PTSD or bipolar disorder; a previous postpartum episode, especially if it was untreated or undertreated, depression, anxiety, or an emotional health problem while pregnant; inadequate social support; marital/partner discord that may or may not escalate to violence; and a family history of anxiety, depression, or other emotional health conditions. Other sources of risk identified by PSI are inadequate support in caring for the baby; financial stress; complications in labor and delivery or breastfeeding; and thyroid imbalance. Also, studies suggest that Hispanic and African American women may be at greater risk, but some of this effect could be due to the socioeconomic disparities and situational stressors.

Infant temperament may likewise influence a mom's likelihood to experience anxiety, depression, or an episode of clinical illness in the perinatal period. Research indicates that mothers who perceive their infants as difficult, irritable, unpredictable, or fussy experience higher levels of PMADs. Reports of more frequent crying or longer episodes of infant crying are associated with increased rates of PMADs. Mothers who perceive infant temperament as a reflection of parenting skills are more likely to experience PMADs (i.e., mothers feel ineffective or inadequate).

Is Anyone NOT at Risk for Pregnancy and Postpartum Anxiety and Depression?

Now that you've read through the laundry list of factors that make some women more likely than others to have a clinical episode of pregnancy or postpartum anxiety, depression, OCD, PTSD, and bipolar disorder, you can begin to see that most women have at least some risk for this condition, and other women have even more. Here's what's important for you to think about if you are worried about your risk. These suggestions are not given as professional advice but mom to mom, and from moms that have experienced postpartum adjustment issues, anxiety, and clinical depression.

First, be your health advocate. Find out what emotional health conditions exist in your family, like anxiety, depression, OCD, or bipolar disorder. If a family member had one of these health conditions, it is much more likely to put you at risk during pregnancy and postpartum, or occur sometime in your life. Be honest with yourself about whether you've ever thought you might have an emotional health condition or had trouble coping with anxiety or depression. Think about how you've managed and responded to other major life changes, like leaving home or getting married. Take the online survey for anxiety and depression symptoms to get an idea of how you're doing.

Second, let your health care providers know your emotional health history and discuss any concerns you may have with them. Then ask to have this information written in your chart so if problems develop, you and your health provider will be able to better decide what to do. If it's recommended that you see a therapist or psychologist, just remember that our specialty is emotional health and stress reduction, which women are more likely to have problems with when they're going through pregnancy and postpartum. As specialists in anxiety and depression, we can help you through talk therapy, and teaching you self-care and other coping skills to better manage your life. Even if you feel ashamed, recall that you are not to blame and that pregnancy and postpartum are the perfect storm of hormones, brain-chemistry changes, and situational stressors that all women experience to some degree, whether they have the baby blues or something more severe, like postpartum anxiety. Know that with the right treatment plan, you'll feel better and like yourself again.

If it's recommended that you see a psychiatrist, go in with an open mind. Most people don't like taking medicine because they think taking it means they're weak or defective. This is not true. If we have an infection, we take an antibiotic so that our health will improve. If we have a broken arm, we get it set. Because in perinatal mood and anxiety disorders, the organ affected is our brain, we may need medicine for it to heal and to function normally again. As Jane Honikman, founder of PSI, says, "It is not your fault. You are not to blame. You will get better."

Finally, if you suspect you are at moderate or high risk for a pregnancy or postpartum condition, educate yourself in advance about where you can find help in your community. Get the names of one or two therapists or a psychiatrist who is familiar with helping women with their reproductive mental health needs, including pregnancy and postpartum. Maybe see one for an initial visit to have them evaluate how you're doing and give you recommendations to lessen your risk. Learn coping skills to manage life change better, like the ones in this book.

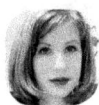

Megan's Mindful-ish Moment: My Unmedicated Life

Disclaimer: I think we all know this, but I have to say it: do not eliminate or reduce any prescribed medication unless under the supervision of a doctor.

When I had postpartum depression and anxiety, a combination of talk therapy, mindfulness practice, and an antidepressant helped me recover. Once my life and mental health had been stable for a couple of years, I decided to look into whether reducing or eliminating the antidepressant was an option. Not only had I learned a lot of strategies for coping with stress, but I was also contemplating having another child in the future. Although out of all antidepressants, mine posed the least risk for an unborn child, I didn't want to take any chances. I also wanted to be sure I could function well, unmedicated, before trying to get pregnant again.

As I reduced my dosage gradually per my doctor's suggestion, I didn't notice any negative effects initially. "Ah ha," I thought, "so I don't need this stuff after all!" I soon realized that it takes a lot more work to stabilize your own moods than letting a pill do it for you.

The first unfamiliar feeling to return after eliminating my antidepressant was annoyance. I found that medicated me and unmedicated me could feel very differently about the same situation. For example, I was still on Zoloft the first time a random stranger asked if Luca's eyelashes were real. "Yes," I answered, baffled by the odd question; after all, my daughter was 2 years old. After a second, I realized the woman was just trying to pay my daughter a compliment. I said thank you on Luca's behalf and went about my day, not giving the encounter a second thought.

By the fourth time this happened, I was no longer taking an antidepressant to temper my reaction. The same question now filled me with irritation. Were they real? What the heck else would they be? "No," I wanted to say, "My daughter cannot possibly leave the house, even to go to the grocery store, without her mascara. She feels positively naked without it!" Or I could have said, "Of course my toddler didn't flinch when I inexplicably approached her eyeball with a pair of tweezers and false lashes. She was doped up with Benadryl!" Or, "Even though the last time I took her to the salon for a simple haircut, she fidgeted so much that the stylist cut herself, I figured, why not? Let's go for the eyelash extensions!" These people might as well have been asking me, "Are you both a sadist and the worst mother ever?" Luckily, my mother had taught me it was impolite to punch people in the throat.

I didn't say any of this out loud, but it was becoming more difficult to be silent about life's habitual irritations. My husband's snoring, the dog's penchant for stealing any food within reach, yet another person remarking on Luca's apparent preference for her daddy—all of this became intolerable. How had I been sailing through life, impervious to these offenses?

A host of other emotions soon rushed in. It became more difficult to remain calm when someone hurt my feelings. I started crying at commercials again. I couldn't watch any episode of *SVU* involving a child. Mindfulness, which had heretofore been little more than a relaxing way to spend a Monday morning, suddenly became a necessity! Gradually, I learned which strategies worked best to deal with which situations. I was able to enjoy the positive emotions, like excitement and optimism, that were amplified along with the negative ones.

Aside from everyone having to get used to the new/old emotional me, everything in my life seemed to be going well. Then, about two years ago, as of this writing, I received some very upsetting news. The content of this news is not my story to tell, but it doesn't matter for our purposes here. The future is going to hold some misfortunes for all of us, whether it be the illness or death of a loved one, the end of a relationship, the loss of a job, or some other traumatic event.

For over three years, my mindfulness skills had helped keep me from sweating the small stuff. But the truth was, I hadn't had to struggle with much "large stuff" since shortly after the birth of my daughter, so I still was unsure if I could remain mindful when confronted with a huge obstacle. When this obstacle appeared, I was initially afraid I would fall apart and that my depression and anxiety would return. I cried a lot. I traveled through all the stages of grief, cycling back to denial a few too many times. Every morning, I woke up feeling okay, only to be crushed again when I remembered that my life had become about five times more complicated than it had been before. So yes, I felt "depressed" and sometimes anxious, but not in the way I'd experienced those feelings postpartum. What I went through was not a clinical episode. It was a natural and normal reaction to what had transpired. I don't think I could have handled it just a couple of years earlier and I didn't initially recognize to what I could credit that change in my coping skills.

The obvious answer would have been the mindfulness I had acquired, but as I was not in a great place to be formally practicing mindfulness, at the time I didn't think I was utilizing those skills. Looking back on it, I kind of understand why that "Footprints in the Sand" poem resonates with so many people. Without realizing it, my mindfulness had transitioned from a *skill set* to a *mindset*, and my mindfulness had essentially carried my grieving self through that difficult time. Also, without the assistance of a 12-step program, I was able to accept what I could not change. Platitudes aren't usually my style, so part of me wants to be cynical and quote the Ani DiFranco lyric:

> I found religion in the greeting card aisle
> And now I know Hallmark was right
> And every pop song on the radio
> Is suddenly speaking to me.

But since I have little interest in being cool these days, identifying with clichés doesn't bother me as much as it would have a decade ago. Instead, it just reminds me how universal my experience was, in stark contrast to the loneliness I felt when going through postpartum depression.

After a couple of months of struggling to wrap my mind around this new world I was living in, I decided to get off my ass and moved on to implement the second line of the serenity prayer. I knew that all the denial and anger and bargaining in the world wasn't going to change everything I wanted it to, so I found the courage to change the things I could. I sat down with Dave, my parents, and everyone who was affected, and made a plan to deal with every damned thing that needed dealing with. And then I went out and got a manicure because I deserved it.

Speaking of self-care, here comes another platitude: every dark cloud has a silver lining. My silver lining, at least in part, is that I never question whether I need to make time for self-care these days. I work hard, I'm extremely busy, and I spend so much time driving that I sometimes feel like a long-haul trucker. So I feel almost zero guilt when I do something for myself.

You may be surprised how little the people you love begrudge you when you do something for yourself because they appreciate how much you do for them. I know Dave mostly appreciates what I do. Luca, on the other hand, told us the other night that she loves the cat more than either of us, but maybe she'll appreciate us more when she's older. At least she'll have to appreciate that we, unlike Mochi, never bit her when she annoyed us.

I haven't forgotten about the wisdom to know the difference between the things you can change and the things you cannot. This is where I see and appreciate my new mindful mindset the most. I can't change the past, and I have little way of knowing what will happen in the future. All any of us can do is do the best we can for ourselves and our families at this moment.

God, grant me the serenity to accept the things I cannot change,

Courage to change the things I can,

And wisdom to know the difference.

Reinhold Niebuhr

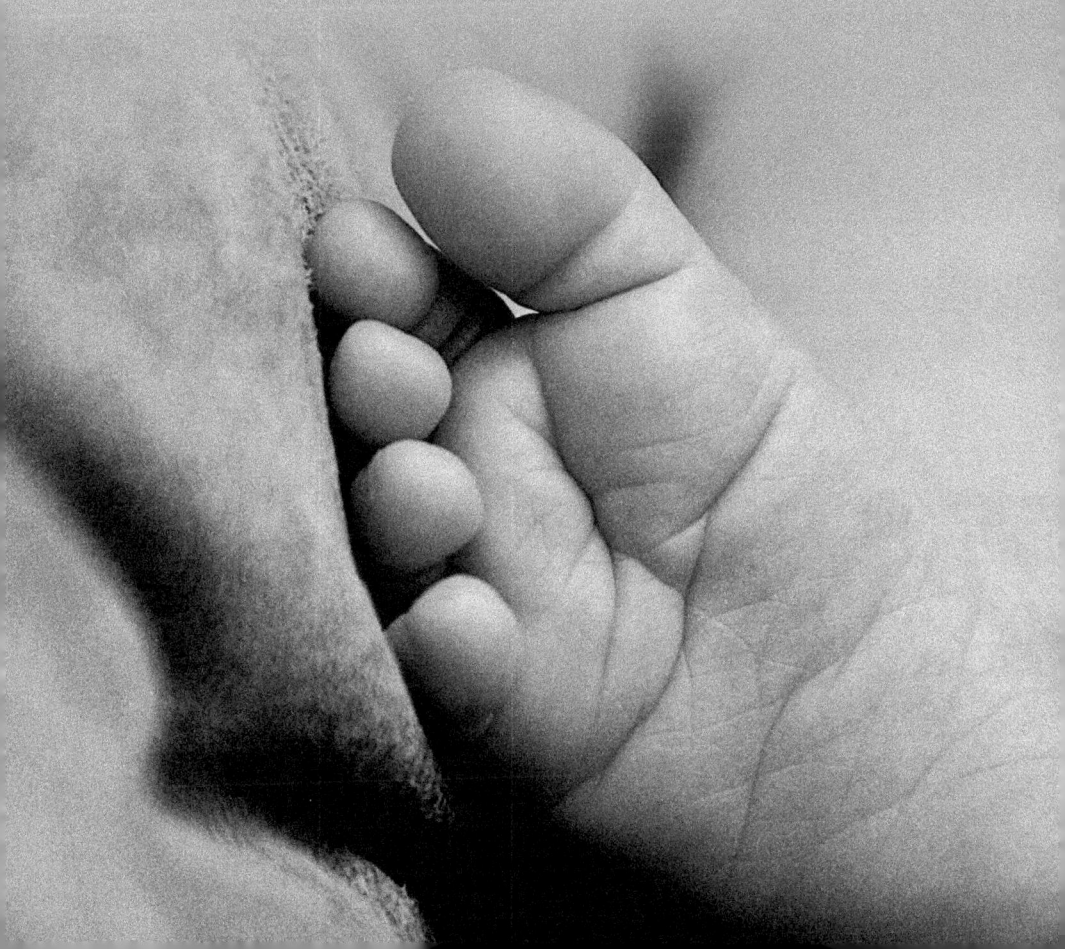

Follow the
GLOW

↑

CHAPTER 3

STRESS REDUCTION

The Fourth Pillar
of Health

To lead a healthy and happy life, you must have a strong foundation. The Four Pillars of Health are nutrition and nourishment; exercise and movement; sleep, rest, and restorative activities; and stress reduction. The first two are often discussed by health experts, and nutrition and exercise programs abound to improve quality of life. Recently, experts have emphasized sleep as important for good health. Arianna Huffington's recent book, which Megan mentioned earlier, is about the health benefits of sleep.

The fourth pillar, stress reduction, is the subject of this book. Although everyone talks about how stress is wrecking our health and ruining our lives, far fewer have committed themselves to pursuing a life of less stress and more ease while resisting the urge to overdo. To lead this kind of life requires that we pay attention to how experience is affecting us and not ignore or minimize our feelings when we are overwhelmed or exhausted. It means noticing when our emotional pitcher is getting empty and taking actions to refill it. Psychologist Wayne Dyer put it this way; "We have become human-doings rather than human beings."

If we are serious about reducing stress, we must practice these skills consistently like we do when we're learning to play an instrument or ride a bike. If we want these skills to become more automatic and accessible, we must make them part of our weekly routine. We must be persistent despite discouraging outcomes and be accepting of gradual but steady progress. It may sound clichéd, but mindfulness is a journey, not a destination. The more we stay the course, the more benefits accrue.

Finally, we must resist cultural expectations that suggest that if we're not accomplishing something and choosing to rest and recharge, we are failing. Adults and children are experiencing anxiety disorders at alarming rates. The on-switch is jammed, and we fear that if we turn it off for a moment, we'll miss out on something. Resisting the status quo is often unsettling, but if we want to improve our health and well-being, it's necessary. In his award-winning book, *The Little Prince*, Antoine de Saint-Exupery said, "It is only through the heart that one can see rightly. What is essential is invisible to the eye."

Stress and Our Experience During Life Transitions

In the last chapter, we talked about how our hormonal and brain chemistry changes, emotional and psychological upheaval, and situational stressors like sleep deprivation make pregnancy and postpartum the perfect storm for stress and dis-ease. This chapter looks at the effects of stress on our minds and bodies, and how easy it is to be carried away, especially during major life transitions, including pregnancy and postpartum. Dr. Alice Domar, who has been a leader in the field of stress reduction for infertility, says that under the right circumstances, like going through IVF and prolonged inability to conceive, our fight-flight reaction may trigger up to 50 times daily. Imagine the vulnerability or risk for stress overload that puts us under while recalling how increased stress can make us more susceptible to anxiety, depression, and issues with our emotional health.

Even when we're not experiencing a major life change, we know that stress impacts all four pillars of health negatively that were discussed in the last chapter. It leads to problems regulating eating behaviors. It affects exercise, physical activity, and our interest in being productive. It frequently results in sleep disturbance and impairs our ability to quiet our mind. In short, it increases physical, mental, and emotional stress symptoms that worsen acute and chronic health conditions.

While the stress reaction was biologically designed to protect us from external threat by signaling alarm and preparing our bodies to fight or flee, it is frequently triggered in today's world by internal thoughts and worries. These "fears" are regarded by the mind and body to be as real as external threats. Chronic prolonged stress may damage our immune system and physical health. Although we know stress is not good for us, many of us are reluctant to slow down for fear of being judged, or judging ourselves.

In mindfulness practice, we say that when we are stressed, we react on autopilot instead of responding with awareness. Our bodies and minds signal danger, as if under attack by an external force.

Likewise, we may not recognize that stress is building until we stop sleeping or start having panic attacks, which can't help but get our attention.

Over time, the effects of stress can be greatly disruptive. As stress increases, it affects all areas of health and well-being—mind, body, heart, and soul. We have increased worry, negative thinking, anxiety, and depression. It lowers self-esteem and self-confidence. It weakens our immune system, decreases energy, disrupts sleep, and disrupts eating and good nutrition. Chronic stress impairs social relationships and increases hostility, resentment, and lack of forgiveness. It diminishes spiritual health and the sense of purpose and contentment with one's life. It may result in feeling less connected to God, a higher power, or the world and others.

If stress can do this under normal circumstances, imagine what it does to a pregnant or postpartum mom when all four pillars of health are already disrupted by what she's going through.

How to Reduce Stress

To reduce stress, we must first acknowledge that it's affecting us and recognize its effects on mind-body health. We must willingly acknowledge when the effects of stress have a negative impact by paying attention to the changes in our bodily sensations, thoughts, and emotions. In mindfulness-based skills practice, this is called the "triangle of awareness." One of the initial skills in stress reduction training is learning to notice our stress profile or how we react under stress.

This profile is different for each of us. Some people will react to stress by becoming agitated, irritated, short-fused, or mean. Others will shut down, get depressed, withdraw, or escape through drugs or food. The same person may react differently depending on what situation triggers it, and alternate between becoming anxious and restless, or depressed and shut down. Monitoring our unique "stress profile," we learn to detect the warning signs that we are overwhelmed and becoming stressed out.

One simple way to begin noticing your stress signals is to keep a stress diary. In the first column, choose a stressful situation from the past week that reached a 5 or above on a scale of 1-10, where 1 is the least amount of stress, and 10 is the most. Describe the situation, other people involved, time of day, and where it happened. Next, write down the bodily sensations you noticed that may include heart racing, palms sweating, dizziness, light-headedness, or stomach in knots. After this column, write down the emotions you felt that could include anger, embarrassment, envy, shame, or any other emotion. In the fourth column, write down whatever thoughts you had.

The object of this exercise is to clarify your stress profile by being honest about what you felt; not making it sound good. Finally, describe what you decided to do to about this situation. If you haven't had a stressful experience this past week, fill out your "Stress Diary Worksheet" with a past stressful incident. You can find the Stress Diary Worksheet and sample stress diary on my website: www.drdianesanford.com.

How Mindfulness-Based Skills Work

Mindfulness-based skills, including the ones in this program, counteract the stress reaction and ease the body's preparedness to fight, flee, or freeze by decreasing the surge of stress hormones, including adrenaline and cortisol. As physical arousal decreases, the body calms down, and thoughts of impending danger decrease. At the moment that we direct our attention from an unpleasant thought, emotion, or bodily sensation to a pleasant or neutral one, we regain control of our ability to respond with a choice instead of reacting with stress.

Remember that most of our stress today is triggered by stressful thoughts instead of saber-toothed tigers. Mental states of worry and regret activate the stress reaction, just like a physical threat. In mindfulness-based skills practice, these unpleasant or negative mental states are called the "tigers within." With mindfulness-based skills, we learn to redirect our attention intentionally away from these tigers within to quiet our minds and bodies.

Mindfulness-based skills enable us to ease physical stress and tension. They have been shown to reduce mental distress and worry, relieve depression and anxiety, and improve immunity and mind-body health. They are the most effective, non-medicinal remedy to reducing stress that currently exists, which is why they are the subject of countless books, including this one. Visit our resource section at the end of this book to learn more.

Megan's Mindful-ish Moment: My Postpartum Experience

I had experienced episodes of anxiety and depression before I was pregnant. I first started to notice them the second semester of my senior year in college, when my self-destructive behavior *du jour* was avoiding writing my senior project. The project was a major endeavor, the supposed culmination of a year of research. It was not one of those 10-page papers I could compose entirely in my head and regurgitate onto the page the night before it was due. I could avoid thinking of the immensity of the challenge and the rapidly approaching deadline for maybe two days at a time, at the end of which I would inevitably dissolve into hysterical fits of crying, hyperventilation, and feeling sure that my life was ending and I would never be happy again. One would think that after a couple of these panic attacks, I would snap out of it, figure out that I was, in fact, not dying, and just do the damn work. But the mind doesn't always work that way, so I would avoid some more, feel worthless and depressed, have another panic attack, rinse and repeat.

Counseling services, I felt, were not an option. Several of my friends and acquaintances had gone there for help and were ultimately sent home to recover. Some would return after a semester, others would transfer, and a couple were neither seen nor heard from again (by myself and my friends, at least). I didn't have the luxury of recuperation. My full-tuition scholarship was good for the standard four-year plan and no more. So I tried to muddle through. I eventually turned in a more-or-less complete senior project, which I did end up working on until the very last minute. I got as good a grade as I could have expected under the circumstances. Despite constant fear that lasted until the moment I walked across the stage and accepted my diploma, I did manage to graduate within the four-year time frame.

For the next couple of years, I worked at a relatively low-stress job. Then I started law school and my problems returned. This time, I did seek help, which did alleviate some of my stress. I didn't get the magic pills that I was halfway hoping for, but I did learn to recognize the symptoms that preceded my panic attacks and succeeded in sometimes preventing their escalation. Life went on: marriage, more jobs, more post-graduate schooling, more therapy. I managed to find a graduate program that wasn't, as one of my former classmates put it, "an exercise in perpetual terror." My husband and I decided to start a family. After almost a year of somewhat lackadaisical attempts, and a few months of making a more concerted effort to conceive, we got pregnant.

My pregnancy was neither a catalog of miserable side effects, nor was it filled with the transcendent joy some mothers describe. It was a normal pregnancy, if normal means by turns thrilling (when I felt the first flutterings of my baby's movement), terrifying (when I fell down the basement stairs and didn't feel her moving for hours), and repulsive (being plagued with uncontrollable farting in the middle of Sephora).

Labor was not everything I hoped it would be. For one thing, I had to be induced before my due date because my blood pressure was "borderline," according to my OB/GYN. What was going on was that I had preeclampsia, which went undiagnosed until I entered the hospital because, before this, I was only exhibiting two out of three of the common symptoms. (Just a few months later, the American College of Obstetrics and Gynecology changed their requirements for a preeclampsia diagnosis.)

For another thing, although I had planned to labor in various birthing positions, induction meant that I couldn't move around without dragging a bunch of tubes and machines behind me. Finally, I had pictured spending my labor watching all three *Anne of Green Gables* movies and possibly the BBC *Pride and Prejudice*, if time allowed, flanked by my husband and my mom. As it turned out, I was too uncomfortable to pay attention to the movies, both because of the contractions and because my hospital bed felt a full foot too short for my 5'11" frame. And when my water finally broke, NO ONE was there. The nurse had gone to retrieve the scary-looking hook for breaking water manually, my parents were in their car on the way back to the hospital, and I'd sent my husband to Sonic for a strawberry-lemon slushie. Woman makes birth plans, God laughs.

When Luca and I came home after delivery, at first, I thought I was sick. I'd just been at the hospital for several days; people always get sick after they've been at hospitals, right? In part because of the preeclampsia, I had gained 52 pounds during pregnancy. Less than two weeks after delivery, I had already shed 43 of them. This was not due to some amazing nutrition and fitness regimen; it was because I could eat next to nothing. I was desperate for food, not so much because I was hungry, but because I knew I needed it to regain my strength and produce breast milk for Luca. Alas, I could keep nothing down.

When I went to my first follow-up visit with my OB/GYN, I was so weak that I couldn't walk from the parking lot to her office without having to rest on a bench (and find a bathroom to be sick in) in between. Because I was unable to eat, my breast milk supply decreased, and Luca's pediatrician told me I had to start supplementing with formula. I had to begin breast pumping several times a day because I couldn't trust myself to produce enough milk to adequately nourish my baby, even for a single feeding. For a while, the severity of my physical symptoms and their accompanying problems eclipsed everything else. Eventually, though, I started to notice the upheaval in my state of mind as well.

I am a great believer in the principle that the universe doesn't give us more than we can handle, but at that time, I wanted to tell the universe to shove it. I was a new mother and couldn't understand how, after two years of desperately wanting this baby, I could be anything but blissfully happy. But I wasn't. Why, after all my research, my devouring of baby books and obsessive nursery outfitting, did I feel so unprepared, so out of control?

I thought I understood lack of sleep. As a student prone to procrastination, I had pulled more all-nighters than I care to remember. So why, when my baby was sleeping soundly, did I startle awake every half hour, filled with terror? Why, with my husband right beside me, with my family larger than it had ever been, did I feel so alone?

I thought I understood pain, too. Since my early teens, I've suffered from GI issues that cause intense stomach cramps. These were frequent enough that it would have been impossible to call in sick to school or work every time I had a "stomachache," so I had to learn to live with the pain while continuing to function normally. I had endured a respectable amount of labor before requesting (okay, more like demanding) the epidural and sustained a Stage 2 tear pushing my daughter's sizeable cranium through my vagina. Getting a tattoo was almost laughably easy. Although I probably couldn't chew off my arm to escape a bear trap, my threshold of pain isn't the lowest. So why was breastfeeding my baby, supposedly such a peaceful, sublime experience, so excruciatingly painful that I spent every minute I wasn't nursing dreading the next feeding?

I thought I understood depression, but I had never experienced such acute feelings of hopelessness, worthlessness, and guilt. I had spent two years talking about how much I wanted a baby, about how I had all this love inside me for which there was no other outlet. So why did I feel suffocated when cudding Luca on my chest? Despite battling almost constant anxieties and catastrophic thoughts, I was cognizant enough to know that this was something more than your everyday case of the baby blues.

As an academically minded individual, on some level, I felt that being well-informed was the solution to all problems and I overloaded my Kindle with account after account of postpartum depression. Although some experiences and symptoms sounded familiar, no story paralleled mine closely enough to comfort me. Reluctantly, I sought help and was referred to Diane.

Diane is one of the warmest, most comforting, most life-affirming people I have ever met. I was in dire need of all her gifts when I came to her on the recommendation of a representative for La Leche League. You know you're in a sorry state when the militant breastfeeding folks tell you to stop worrying about nursing and take care of yourself!

Sometimes mindfulness practice is all a person needs to relieve stress and anxiety. At other times, it needs to be coupled with more drastic intervention to be most effective. This was the case with me. To overcome my postpartum depression and anxiety, I first needed Zoloft and talk therapy. It took a few months of getting stabilized before Diane even mentioned mindfulness practice, but it proved to be the final piece of the puzzle in my recovery. I began to practice regularly with a group of other women, dubbed "The Mindful Moms" and led by Diane. We did many of the exercises discussed in this book and shared our experiences, both with mindfulness and in our day-to-day lives.

It was important for me to carve out space in my schedule dedicated to self-care and stress reduction. For a couple of hours every Monday morning, I allowed myself to let go of worries, stop making to-do lists in my head, and give my attention to the present moment. In addition to the formal practice I did in class and at home, I learned how to practice informally. Sometimes just noticing tension in my body and following my breath is enough to alleviate stress.

Mindfulness helped with my periods of insomnia, too. Soon after I began practicing mindful meditation, I was able to stop taking the Ambien my doctor had prescribed. I still experience the occasional difficulty falling and staying asleep, but listening to one of Diane's guided meditations or following my breath while silently repeating my mantra at bedtime really helps calm my "monkey mind." And with mindfulness, I don't have to worry about any bizarre side-effects!

For a couple of years after Luca was born, I continued to take Zoloft, albeit in a lower dosage than I did in the beginning. Since then, I have been able to eliminate that as well. I still have therapy sessions with Diane, but I need fewer of them now than I once did. Mindfulness, however, has only grown more important to me.

Diane has reminded me more than once that mindfulness is best learned in periods of relative calm. Then, when stressful situations do arise, we can call upon what we have learned to help us through those times, which I have done on many occasions over the past five years. Now I am confident that, when and if Dave and I have another child, I will have all the resources and tools I need in my mental health arsenal to have a much better experience than I did the first time around.

I wanted to share my experience with PPD to assure other women who may feel the way I did that they are not alone. I know that it can be difficult to ask for help or admit having PPD because there is still such a stigma attached to mental illness. Despite the number of celebrity testimonials surrounding PPD, women afflicted with it are still misunderstood and maligned. Seeking to explain how some mothers could harm their children, the popular media is quick to speculate that PPD is the cause. Misleading information like this may prevent those of us who love and want to protect our babies from seeking treatment, fearing guilt by association.

Like the vast majority of mothers experiencing PMADs, I never dreamed of harming my child. Unlike Brooke Shields, I never felt the irrational urge to toss my baby out the window. I did, however, occasionally fantasize that I was her babysitter and could return her to her real, competent, and appropriately grateful parents at the end of the night.

I mourned all the things I felt I could no longer do. The observation that "life will never be the same" stopped sounding like the beginning of an exciting adventure and started sounding like the beginning of extremely lengthy prison term.

But to be perfectly honest, I didn't especially *want* to do those things that becoming a parent rendered prohibitive. Sure, I couldn't drink so much on a Friday night as to make myself hungover and useless for the remainder of the weekend. But I had found nine months without a drop of alcohol to be surprisingly easy, and drinking no longer seemed mandatory at all social functions, as it had seemed in my twenties. And, no, Dave and I couldn't pick up and leave on vacation at a moment's notice. But we never actually did that pre-Luca; we always had work, school, pets, and other obligations that forced us to plan all holidays well in advance. Other things, like leisurely brunches and afternoon sex, are admittedly a bit harder to manage but still possible on occasion.

Leaving the house did seem like a major production for a while— stock diaper bag with diapers, wipes, changing pad, burp rags, blankets, toys, snacks, changes of clothes, Swiss Army knife, flare gun, etc.; dress baby in non-stained clothing, invariably complete with matching hat, even if it's 100 degrees outside and cute shoes, even though baby cannot walk; strap baby into cumbersome infant carrier and attach it to car seat base; then drive to destination only to realize you have forgotten to put on your pants. But before we knew it, we had a fully ambulatory little person capable of carrying her own tools of distraction and ever-more-willing to sit on a large public toilet seat with minimal complaint. Now Luca is quite the conversationalist (if you're into princesses and superheroes) and we can take her almost anywhere. Sometimes, though, I do miss those infant years, even with all their attendant needs.

Life never would be the same, but as I progressed through recovery, it started to feel more like the adventure I'd hoped it would be. Somehow, I had found the courage inside myself to say, "Something isn't right, and I need help to fix it." I had admitted that my baby did make me feel trapped, that I didn't feel that "maternal instinct" everyone said came so naturally, that I feared I had made a terrible mistake. Fortunately, my support system assured me that I wasn't alone in feeling the way I did, that things could get better, that I wasn't a bad mother. Eventually, I started to believe what they were saying.

Luca is a joy and a blessing, and I am so glad that I didn't sleepwalk through the first few years of her life in depression. Oddly enough, the minute I admitted to myself and others that my life felt all wrong was the minute things started to turn around until eventually, everything turned out all right. The universe may never give us more than we can handle, but nobody said we need to handle it alone.

A Short History of Mindfulness-Based Skills

Buddha and other teachers developed mindfulness to teach human beings how to suffer less and live better. It is said that when Buddha was born, the wise men predicted that he would either become a great leader or a great teacher. To ensure that he would become a great leader, the king made him stay within the palace walls so he would live and not know suffering existed.

For 15 years, Buddha never left the palace, but when he turned 16, he asked his charioteer, who was said to be a guardian angel, to take him to see the world outside. On these three consecutive days, he encountered people who were ill, aging, and dead. Disturbed by what he'd seen, he dedicated his life to discovering how to end human suffering.

First, he studied in a monastery where he learned meditation, compassion, and contemplative thought, but grew restless and left after several years. Next, he became an ascetic, wandering the country without any possessions, relying on the charity of others for food, clothes, and shelter when needed. One day, tired and near starvation, he went to drink from a stream and saw his reflection. Appearing worn and much older than his years, he thought; "Certainly this can't be the path to enlightenment and what God wants for me."

After restoring his health, he stopped and meditated under a Bodhi tree for 40 days and nights. During this time, he was visited by many dreams and thoughts that kept alternating between pleasant, neutral, and unpleasant experiences. Whatever happened, he let it arise in his mind and then go away. From this experience, he learned that all thoughts, feelings, and bodily sensations are temporary and pass in time. To end suffering, we must retrain our minds to be aware and allow whatever happens to happen without trying to cling to pleasure or avoid pain.

If we follow Buddha's example and learn mindfulness skills, it can offset some of the painful, unavoidable circumstances we experience. While there is no way around sleep loss, many of the moms who work with me use these skills to deal with insomnia and their overly active and fearful minds that keep them awake, even when the baby sleeps. When practiced consistently, mindfulness skills ease stress and worry in our daily lives and periods of mind-body upheaval, like pregnancy and postpartum.

Overview of My Stress Less, Live Better Mindfulness-Based Program

If women are caregivers in general, then new moms qualify for the label "ultimate" caregivers because they devote 24/7 of their time to making certain their infant's needs are met, often at the cost of their own health and well-being. My program was developed with women in mind, who often seek my counsel when they're going through life changes: mind, body, and spirit. About half the women I teach come to see me for factors related to childbearing: having a baby, experiencing a pregnancy loss, having fertility issues, experiencing a complicated pregnancy, or having a traumatic birth experience. The other half of them usually show up around peri-menopause or menopause, when life changes and hormonal influences collide again, becoming too much to handle on their own.

Although many women and men I see in my practice may have clinical anxiety, obsessive-compulsive disorder (OCD), posttraumatic stress disorder (PTSD), depression, or other mood conditions, they also lead exceptionally busy lives. They are articulate, bright, educated, and involved with their families and their communities. They are not the people you expect to show up in a psychologist's office except that they are suffering mentally, emotionally, and physically in ways that have become unbearable. Most realize that they want to feel better, but nothing they do or have tried is helping, so they seek professional advice.

Because their lives are already so full, initially they can't imagine adding mindfulness skills practice to their routine. Likewise, they don't believe that something so simple will ease their distress and improve their health. They look at me skeptically, thinking (perhaps you are too) that I am offering some new-age mumbo jumbo that can't possibly work, even though evidence-based studies indicate that it does. In a rush to feel better, they want something that will reduce their depression and anxiety quickly and effortlessly. When I explain that learning mindfulness skills is simple but not easy, and requires persistent effort and regular practice, their eyes glaze over. In their desperation, they consent to practice in small, attainable ways. As they do, it works if they keep persisting in making these changes.

After attending one of my classes, one of my students, who is a humorist, wrote an article in her weekly column in a local magazine in which she gave me one of my biggest compliments ever.

I get migraines, and my doctor suggested I
de-stress by learning some mindfulness
techniques, which is code for "learn how to
calm yourself down before you stroke out."
That's how I found myself at Dr. Diane
Sanford's Midwest Mind-Body Health Center.
Now, I have always scoffed, actually mocked
any kind of meditation as being "fluffy."
You know, only for people who wear hemp and
eat flaxseeds. I was wrong. The one hour I
spent hanging my thoughts on clouds and
watching them float away was one of the most
relaxing I've had in months. It ranks right up
there with my usual form of relaxation:
reality TV, a diet Coke, and peanut M&M's.
(Hannum, 2015)

Mindfulness in Five Simple Steps

To accommodate my students' needs for a way to practice these skills that were not time-consuming and could be incorporated more easily into their daily lives, I came up with dividing the skills I'd learned from many teachers into five skillsets. Wanting to make them easy to remember, each starts with the letter "S," which made them easier for me to recall too. The five mindfulness-based skillsets that are discussed in my class and this book are: Simply Breathe; Soothe Your Body; Savor the Moment; Settle Your Thoughts, and Self-Compassion Always.

Each skillset has a different focus of attention, although all of them require directing your attention to the present moment on purpose with self-compassion, which is the definition of mindfulness. The goal of each of the five skillsets is to learn to direct your attention intentionally so that you can stress less and live better by not dwelling on unpleasant worries about the future or regrets about the past. Also, each skillset has an underlying intention or goal that's being taught in order, where the previous exercises are the foundation for the next set. Both formal and informal means of practicing each skillset are given.

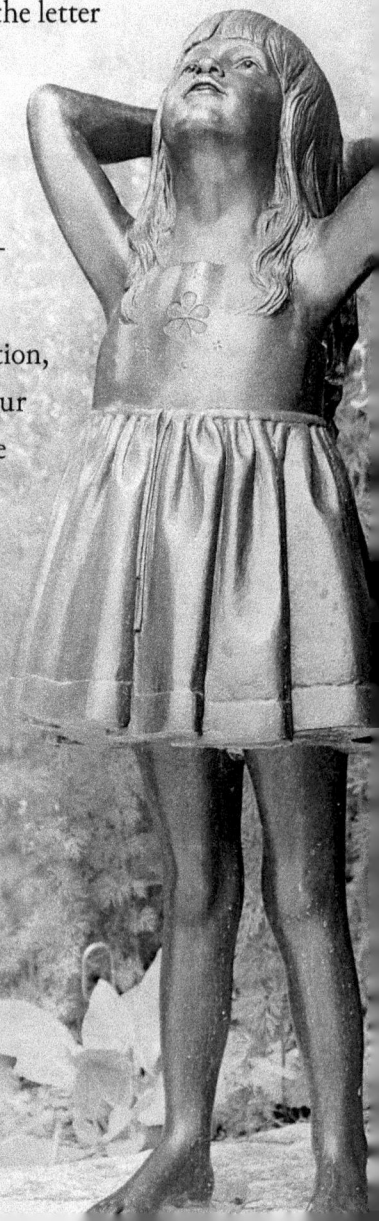

With Simply Breathe, you learn to notice your experience as it's occurring by focusing on your breath. Soothe Your Body is about paying attention to what's happening in the present moment through body awareness. Savor the Moment involves sensing the experience we're having with all five senses: sight, sound, touch, taste, and smell. In Settle Your Thoughts, the intention is not clinging to thoughts or emotions but letting them come and go. Finally, Self-Compassion Always is about accepting yourself with self-compassion rather than self-criticism, which is perhaps the most challenging skill to practice. Each skillset is presented in a separate chapter with exercises in the book and online for you to practice.

When to Seek Professional Help

Because expecting and new moms can progress quickly from normal adjustment reactions to a clinical condition, here are some guidelines for when to seek professional help. First, here are some warning signs that stress is building and may become more than you can handle on your own.

* Trouble falling asleep or staying asleep

* Overeating or eating too little

* Physical symptoms including headache, gastrointestinal problems, and muscle tension

* Irritability or being short-fused

* Fatigue and lack of energy

* Increase in negative thinking and worry

* Feeling overwhelmed and anxious

* Feeling down, weepy, or sad

❋ Decrease in joy and life satisfaction

❋ Being inattentive and forgetful

All these changes are normal when your mind and body are stressed by short-term or prolonged stress, and everyone will experience some of these problems some of the time. What's most important is to learn to recognize when you are becoming stressed, or when your stress is increasing, and how to cope in ways that preserve and may improve your health and well-being.

Here are some guidelines to indicate that you may be starting to experience a clinical episode of depression or anxiety and what to do:

❋ If you've experienced mood or anxiety symptoms that are interfering with your ability to care for yourself or your child.

❋ If mood and anxiety symptoms are getting worse, not better, over 2 weeks.

❋ If you're experiencing mood and anxiety changes that are bothering you and starting to impact your confidence and esteem.

❋ If sleep disturbance and anxiety over sleeping are becoming moderately to severely distressing.

❋ If you've noticed moderate changes in attention and concentration, and you seem to be getting more confused and distracted.

❋ If you are moderately to severely agitated and over-whelmed.

❋ If you are moderately to severely irritable and upset with others, specifically your spouse or partner.

* If other people are concerned about how much anxiety and mood changes are affecting you.

* If you are having recurrent thoughts of escaping your life by running away or other means.

* If you have thoughts of harming yourself, your baby, or others.

* If mood and anxiety symptoms have gotten stronger than a 5 on a 10-point scale for two weeks, call your health provider and get checked out.

As a psychologist, these are the problems I see when an expecting or new mom comes for treatment because she's having what I call a "pile up" and her stress switch is jammed and can't be turned down or off.

Again, moderate to severe diagnosable clinical conditions are most likely to require a combination of therapy, medication, and support for the mom to recover fully. The sooner treatment begins, the quicker she can get better and be the person she wants to be for herself and family.

Once a mom's brain has calmed down, a mindfulness skills-building like my Stress Less, Live Better curriculum is very helpful to recovery and relapse prevention. However, initial treatment for PMADs should focus on the mom's present situation, helping her lessen stress through self-care and having others support her if available, and getting her symptoms, including sleep disturbance, anxiety, and depression to settle down and, ideally, go away.

If you are seeing a psychiatrist, psychologist, or therapist who wants to discuss your childhood, or is not directly addressing the pregnancy and postpartum factors that are causing you to have problems, stop seeing them. Perinatal mood and anxiety disorders

(PMADs) are an acute health condition that requires care based on your immediate circumstances. Likewise, if you suspect that you or someone you know is having an episode of postpartum psychosis that usually starts with extreme sleeplessness; mania or over-activity; mounting confusion; and overabundance of energy, speeded up speech and behavior; and excessively strange thoughts and ideas, take them to the ER or their doctor right away. Postpartum psychosis is an URGENT medical condition that can deteriorate rapidly, and in rare cases, lead to maternal suicide or infant death because of the mom's delusional and disordered thinking.

If you want to learn more about what PMADs look like and how they progress, go to PSI's website (www.postpartum.net) or consult expert Karen Kleiman's website (www.postpartumstress.com) for educational information and clinical resources.

Today was a
good day,
How. are you?

CHAPTER 4

THE STRESS LESS, LIVE BETTER PROGRAM
for Pregnancy, Postpartum, and Early Motherhood

The Stress Less, Live Better program for expecting and new moms combines, self-care, the Four Pillars of Health, and the 5 Simple Steps introduced in the last chapter. While many pregnant moms go out of their way to practice good health habits during pregnancy, these tend to fall apart postpartum when the mom's attention is directed to her newborn and away from herself. However, it's equally important to maintain healthy mind-body habits postpartum because to take care of someone else, you need to take care of yourself.

If that's not reason enough to make your health and well-being a priority, then think about this. Starting in the 1950s, researchers in developmental psychology began studying the impact of maternal well-being and health on their newborns, toddlers, and children. These studies consistently showed that moms with depression, anxiety, and emotional-health issues were more likely to have children with cognitive, social, and emotional impairments. These children may have a lower IQ, specific learning disabilities, and problems in school. They are at increased risk for behavioral issues, like being disruptive or inattentive and hyperactive. Because of their insecure attachment or bonding to their moms, these infants and children had more trouble with social interactions and forming or maintaining close interpersonal relationships. There was also a greater risk for child abuse and neglect among these moms towards their infants.

So, if you can't practice good physical and emotional health habits for yourself, do it for your baby. For the past several decades, women have been cautious and concerned about experiencing a healthy pregnancy, but that's just the start of our motherhood journey. Now, we must learn to make our health and wellbeing a priority because if we don't, everyone will suffer.

Choosing Healthier, More Effective Coping Skills

Although it is true that stress increases during pregnancy, postpartum, and early motherhood, awe do not have to resort to less healthy, more immediately gratifying ways of coping such as overeating, drinking too much, overworking, smoking more, and participating in other addictive behaviors. We can learn through the practice of mindful stress reduction to choose options that enhance health instead. In mindfulness practice, we say that we become aware of reacting on autopilot and reverting to our conditioned ways of soothing ourselves rather than responding with choice. This doesn't mean that using these skills makes us feel better or relieves stress immediately. Instead, over time, these mindful stress-reduction strategies are more likely to reduce stress and improve our mind-body health. Regular practice of mindfulness strategies can boost immunity, improve mood, and increase wellbeing by decreasing anxiety, depression, and worry.

How does this work? The idea behind mindful stress reduction is that we are constantly frightening ourselves with worries about the future or regrets about the past, and that this results in stressful and unpleasant thoughts, feelings, and bodily sensations. By learning to re-inhabit the present moment and focus our attention intentionally on what's going on, we can reduce the stress of these worries and regrets. Because, as human beings, we can't think about more than one thing at a time (though many people think they can), our minds are occupied with what's happening now instead of the future or past. This helps us to feel better and more capable of dealing with present moment stress and challenges, and not stealing the energy and strength caregivers need to keep going.

Unlike our caveman ancestors, who had to run from the saber-toothed tiger to stay alive, these days, we are frightened primarily by what we think about. Our bodies react to them by producing an increase in cortisol, adrenaline, and other stress hormones as they would if we were physically threatened. Unfortunately, once the stress reaction triggers, it is difficult to turn off and we end up in a constant state of alarm. Most of my clients' anxiety and depression are fueled by these worries from years of conditioning.

I developed my Stress Less, Live Better program for moms and people with busy, active lives who frequently commented on how stress was wrecking their lives, but didn't have time to practice yoga or meditate for 45 minutes twice a day. I wanted to make the mindfulness skills I had learned over the past 15 years easy to understand and practice. That's how Stress Less, Live Better came about. Some exercises are short and last about 5 minutes, while others take up to 15 minutes. They are designed to become part of your daily routine easily, without much fuss. Likewise, you can use many of the activities that already occur in your day by learning how to approach them more mindfully.

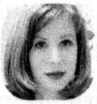

Megan's Mindful-ish Moment: First-World Problems

First-World Problems

Mark Twain once said, "I am a very old man and have suffered many misfortunes, most of which never occurred." Diane likes to cite this fairly well-known quote because it speaks to our tendency to get carried away with our negative thoughts and become convinced that imagined threats are real. Slightly less familiar but in the same vein is this Thomas Jefferson quote:

> There are... gloomy & hypochondriac minds, inhab-
> itants of diseased bodies, disgusted with the present,
> & despairing of the future; always counting that the
> worst will happen, because it may happen. To these
> I say, "How much pain have cost us the evils which
> have never happened!"

How much indeed. I would be a bit more charitable toward these "gloomy and hypochondriac minds" and simply call them "worriers."

There seems to be a pervasive feeling in our culture that experiencing anxiety over someone or something is compulsory if we care about that person or issue. Being a parent is almost synonymous with being a worrier. To some people, worry can be like a badge of honor, showing what a caring and empathetic person you are. But worry has no practical value to anyone. It is unhealthy for you and does nothing to help the person or problem that is the focus of your worry. Merely fretting about climate change is not going to reduce fossil fuel emissions or repair the ozone layer. Worrying about your child will not shield him from all the world's harms. Worry is only helpful when it's an impetus for positive action; unfortunately, it rarely is.

I'm not suggesting that it is possible to stop worrying entirely; it is natural to be concerned about people and issues that are important to us. The problem comes in when we start to get bent out of shape over something that simply *does not matter*. That's when we need a reality check to put things in perspective. I like to utilize an exercise I call the "First-World Problems Test."

I recently became aware that some people have never heard the term "First-World Problem" or "Champagne Problem" (not to be confused with "drinking problem"). I don't have an official definition for this phenomenon, but this is how I have come to understand it. There are basic human needs, such as food, shelter, and general bodily safety. Then there are somewhat less basic but still important human rights like sanitation, healthcare, education, the pursuit of happiness, the freedom to love whom we choose, et cetera. When these needs and rights are threatened, that constitutes a problem.

To call something a First-World problem is not to say that violations of needs and rights only occur in developing countries. Nor does it mean that a breach of human rights or needs is the only thing that qualifies as a problem. Loved ones die, people lose their jobs and their homes, marriages fail; all of these would qualify as problems, no matter where you live. The concept that something can be a First-World problem is just a tongue-in-cheek reminder that, somewhere, people are still starving and genocide is happening, so don't have a meltdown if someone cuts you off in traffic or your kid doesn't make the cheerleading squad. In the grand scheme of things, most of our so-called "problems" are not that big of a deal and not worth compromising our emotional wellbeing over.

When I find myself worrying or getting upset about something, I put it to the First-World-Problem Test. If it's a First-World problem, I endeavor to let it go. I bought a pair of shoes for full price last week and now they're 50% off? First-World problem. Has Luca failed to meet some arbitrary developmental milestone by some arbitrarily set age? First-World problem. Husband falls asleep in church *again*? Annoying, but still a First-World problem.

There are various subsets of First-World problems, such as white-girl problems, to which I occasionally fall victim as well. I once spent an entire afternoon researching at-home hair removal lasers to determine if they would be suitable for ridding myself of unwanted "baby hairs" along my hairline, then wondering whether I would ultimately, like Kim Kardashian, regret that I removed these hairs in the first place as the procedure had rendered my face less "youthful." Call me a vain, frivolous person with too much time on my hands, but at least I eventually employed the First-World problem test. If not for that, I might be here looking five years older and being $500 poorer.

Simplify Your Life

In addition to employing the First-World-Problem test and "letting it go," another way to reduce stress is to simplify your life. Some stressors in life are unavoidable. Maybe your job is stressing you out, but you have to make money somehow. Maybe your family is driving you crazy, but it would be wrong to run out to "pick up some milk" and never come back. Some stressors, though, are completely avoidable and unnecessary.

For several summers, I gave myself fits over sunless tanners. One was too expensive, while another faded too fast. One was too orange, another too streaky. Twice a week, I spent 20 minutes sloughing off dead skin with some loofah and scrub, 20 minutes applying self-tanner, and 20 minutes walking around naked waiting for it to dry. Then there was the daily maintenance with "gradual" tanning lotions. I was always trying to keep my palms, toes, and fingernails from turning orange. And why was it that I felt I needed a faux glow to look good in white, yet the very product that allowed me to wear white also left stains, changing all this clothing from white into something more akin to yellow?

Eventually, I had to take a step back and consider why I thought I needed a tan, and why the natural color of my skin wasn't good enough. Sure, I could look back on my childhood in the 80s and 90s. At that time, having a bitchin' tan signaled health and attractiveness rather than cancer and premature aging. The other kids in elementary school always teased me for having fair skin. But why should something that happened almost 30 years ago affect my decisions now? There should be no shame in the natural color of one's skin, whatever it may be.

Faux-tanning wasn't just a body-image issue for me; it was also a lifestyle problem, a hassle, and a stressor. I decided to simplify my life and ditch the gels, lotions, and spray-booths, and it has been nothing but a relief. Currently, I'm happy being a "pale princess" and, thus far, no 9-year-olds have called me "Casper" or accused me of never playing outside.

I realize that, here and elsewhere, I tend to use examples that relate to physical appearance, beauty products, retail therapy, and other stereotypically "female" interests. Dilemmas concerning these areas are especially useful to use as examples of First-World issues not worthy of worry because, to most people, they are so obviously superficial. This is not to suggest that people who identify as more feminine have cornered the market on trivial pseudo-problems. The sentiment of the First-World problem can apply to any non-mandatory, possibly stress-inducing activity: keeping up with the neighbors, competitive coupon-clipping, volunteering for every event at your child's school, overindulging in social media, or playing any video or online game that requires routine maintenance. Remember when everyone was running around, chasing after imaginary Pokemon? Trust me, you don't "gotta catch 'em all."

Simplify Your Pregnancy and New Motherhood

Having a child can make you reexamine your priorities in a positive way, but preparing for the arrival of your little one can also be a lot like planning a wedding in the sense that it lends itself to obsessing over truly silly and insignificant things. If you are currently pregnant, I can advise you from experience to not go overboard in planning your baby's nursery. Buy the absolute necessities and then worry about everything else if you have the time and inclination. Buy what appeals to you, because your baby is not going to care and this will probably be the last time you will have complete control over the appearance of your child's room.

The same keep-it-simple rule applies when purchasing a baby's clothing. People who know me are going to laugh, but I've learned from my mistakes, so take my word on this. Many new moms or moms-to-be find it irresistible to buy fancy outfits for newborn babies, but I recommend resisting the temptation as much as possible. It will soon become abundantly clear that function is everything when your little angel starts peeing, pooping, and vomiting on everything within range. Even with the multiple daily wardrobe changes that were necessary with Luca, she grew so quickly that we ended up with onesies that she only wore once. By all means, buy cute, impractical things for special occasions, but for the rest of the time, take it easy on yourself.

Sorry to say, the fashionable cut or clean lines of a garment aren't going to make your newborn baby look any less like a sack of potatoes. (The most adorable and charming sack of potatoes ever, but a sack of potatoes nonetheless.) Think about how your clothes look when you've slept in them and magnify that by ten; then you will have an idea of how well Luca's outfits presented in the first year of her life. Things change a bit when your baby starts to walk. You can start to dress her in the latest fashions if you are so inclined, but before you know it, your toddler will start having definitive opinions regarding what she wants to wear, and it will be time to employ the First-World-Problems test. Ask yourself, is this a battle worth fighting? Sure, the lavender tutu with a bunny tail attached paired with the fluorescent yellow shirt may put your teeth on edge, but insisting she change now may upset the karmic balance and give you less influence over some other, more important choices she might make, such as whether or not to share her toys. Besides, if you're anything like me, you've witnessed your partner making outfit choices for your child that are every bit as questionable as those she would make for herself.

Similar to the way he will exert his will over dressing, your child will also form interests and play preferences surprisingly early, so try not to buy a lot of age-inappropriate toys for "when he gets a little older." While he is a baby who can barely hold his head up, you may dream of the day when he is zipping around in a motorized mini-Ferrari. But do you want to let it sit around in your garage or basement for four years until he's old enough to use it? You may find that by that time, he would infinitely prefer a tractor or be content to remain a passenger for a few more years. In that case, you will be kicking yourself for spending all that money in the first place and may run the risk of foisting the toy upon your child with too much enthusiasm, which will probably make him even less disposed to play with it.

Finally, if you want to simplify your pregnancy and new motherhood, refrain from making any huge life changes during your pregnancy, if possible. You may have little idea of how having a baby will affect you, but you can be sure that you will be exhausted. The impending arrival of their babies makes some women determined to get all their ducks in a row (and not just the rubber variety). There is a difference between being prepared and attempting to achieve all your life's goals in between increasingly frequent pee breaks.

Major life changes may include changing careers, moving, or beginning any large-scale home improvements. I sometimes watch home renovation or house hunting shows, as this type of programming, although designed for adults, would still be appropriate for a kindergartner to see. Have you ever noticed how often these programs feature women who are about eight months pregnant, and how often said pregnancy is cited as the reason for a new and improved home? These couples must be thinking, "Hey, we are about to embark on one of life's most magical yet harrowing journeys! Let's hire someone to destroy our kitchen so we can't use it for three months!"

Another major change that no pregnant couple should take lightly is the decision to adopt a pet, especially a high-maintenance one. When I was three months pregnant, someone (okay, it was me) had the brilliant idea to adopt a puppy. Dave and I had just lost our beloved dog, Anjin, to bone cancer. Although Dave would have probably preferred a longer grieving period, I persuaded him that there was no better time to get a new family dog. I reasoned that provided we were diligent owners, said dog would be well-trained by the time our baby arrived, and who knew when we would again have the time to train a puppy? Then the new pet and the newer baby could grow up together. Dave and I both had fond memories of our childhood family pets, so two days after Christmas 2012, we drove to the shelter and came home with a 12-week-old Shiba Inu.

These dogs have been internet darlings since the puppy cam videos of 2008, and the breed has since become further popularized by the ubiquitous "doge" meme. Although Shibas are the most popular dog breed in Japan, one will seldom find them in shelters in this country, so I felt very fortunate that Kitsu was available to adopt. If we had done our research more thoroughly, Dave and I would have learned that, though adorable, Shiba Inus are notoriously stubborn and often too smart for their own good.

Most of you are aware that morning sickness and extreme sensitivity to smells are two of the most common side effects of pregnancy. I have never been fond of scooping poop, but nothing compares to the unpleasantness of cleaning up after a puppy that has just had explosive diarrhea all over the kitchen floor, especially when one is already prone to nausea. On the bright side, with all the potty accidents and crying in the night, Kitsu was providing

Dave and me with plenty of practice for the months and years ahead. Dogs and cats are a lot like toddlers who never grow up.

Despite passing two obedience courses with flying colors, Kitsu was not the perfectly trained dog I had hoped she would be by the time Luca was born. Like teething babies, puppies will chew on anything they can get their mouths on, and Kitsu had already chewed giant bald patches in the living room rug. She was jealous and resentful when Luca arrived and displaced her as the baby of the family. The dog got her revenge by chewing up anything that belonged to Luca. Bottle nipples were her favorite treat, but blankets, stuffed animals, and a plethora of plastic stacking toys also felt her wrath. Once Luca started to toddle around, often holding some snack, Kitsu was always angling to steal the proverbial candy from the baby.

Reflecting on Luca and Kitsu's lack of affinity for one another, I considered the fact that I had been about 3 years old when our family acquired Molly, the polydactyl tabby cat I remember so fondly. The cat my parents had when I was an infant and toddler, a black Persian with an irresistibly fluffy, pullable tail, had despised me and hid under a bed whenever I came near. When Luca was 3, she got her special kitten. She and the now 2-year-old Mochi are thick as thieves. Like Molly, Mochi is big, friendly, and fairly tolerant of Luca's sometimes overexuberant affection, and while he participates in tea parties, he draws the line at being dressed in a tutu.

Kitsu and Luca eventually declared a ceasefire and stopped competing for food. Now Luca loves to feed Kitsu french fries, which, let's face it, are far tastier than most of the snacks the pooch managed to filch during Luca's toddler years. Kitsu much prefers Dave's company to anyone else's, so she doesn't mind playing second fiddle to Mochi in Luca's heart.

Sometimes I look around and lament the havoc my child and pets have wreaked on the house. There are chocolate smears on the sofa cushions and toys scattered on the floor, most of the furniture legs have been visibly chewed, there's fur everywhere, and every so often, I hear the sound of someone's paw knocking something breakable off a shelf. "This is why we can't have nice things," I tell Luca. But that's okay. It's a First-World Problem.

📄 EXERCISE

The Comfort-Stone Exercise

The first exercise I do in class is called The Comfort Stone. I named it this to make a positive statement about what the stone is used for rather than calling it a "worry" stone. I want moms to know that they're relying on their comfort stones to help them calm their minds and bodies when they're uncomfortable and distressed. I often give clients stones for their child or a good friend who may be going through a rough time. I am always surprised at how much people and their loved ones benefit from having the stone and how much it truly helps.

The first step is finding a stone. Once you have it, you're ready. I use the ones you'd put in a vase from the Dollar Store. Start by placing the stone in your hand and closing your other hand over it or holding it in your hands to your heart. Close your eyes or keep them open, and take three deep breaths, slowly breathing in to the count of three through your nose and out to the count of three through your mouth.

Then begin to think about someone you love or a pleasant memory that you recall. The idea is for the stone to remind you of pleasant feelings instead of fear or worry. If you can't recall someone or some experience that brings you pleasant feelings, then say your

ABCs or count to one hundred or think of something else that isn't stressful. Mindfulness teachers say that all experience is divided into being pleasant, neutral, or unpleasant. In this exercise, we are focusing on pleasant or neutral feelings to reduce stress and increase comfort.

Spend the next few minutes thinking about your loved one, or a pleasant memory or experience. Recall it in as much detail as you can. Visualize it. Notice any other sensory experiences associated with it, like the warmth of the sun on your face or the scent of autumn leaves burning. When your mind wanders, and it will, bring your attention back to imagining your loved one or a pleasant experience. Then take three more deep breaths in and out, and if your eyes are closed, open them. You can find a guided version of this exercise at www.drdianesanford.com.

Overview of Stress Less and Live Better: 5 Simple Steps to Ease Anxiety, Worry, and Self-Criticism

As a mom, there isn't much time in the day for your stress reduction. So, here is an overview of my five skill sets with an exercise for each that you can do in five minutes or less. It is more important to practice regularly and at consistent intervals than not practice because it's too time-consuming and you have other things that must get done. I suggest you practice one of the following exercises two or three days a week to start. The next chapter of this book describes each of these skill sets in greater detail with additional exercises and questions for reflection. You can also go to www.drdianesanford.com, click on Resources, and follow me for guided exercises.

General Guidelines for Mindfulness Practice

Before reviewing each of the 5 Simple Skills in the next five chapters, let's discuss the guidelines for practicing mindfulness-based skills. Recall that mindfulness is defined as "being aware of the present moment on purpose with self-compassion or non-judgment." In addition to directing our attention to the moment we're in, and the thoughts, feelings, and bodily sensations we're having, I encourage students to have a curious and accepting attitude towards themselves, whatever happens as they practice the 5 Simple Skills.

Let me give you an example. When I'm teaching a class, students get nervous practicing the exercises because they think they're not doing them right or perfectly. I explain to them that there is no right or wrong way to do these exercises because the point is to be aware of your experience. They figure out how to treat themselves with self-compassion and acceptance, not comparison and rejection. Remember, the goal of mindfulness is to become more aware of yourself and notice what stirs you up as well as what settles you. It is not a competition. All it requires is a willing spirit and an open mind.

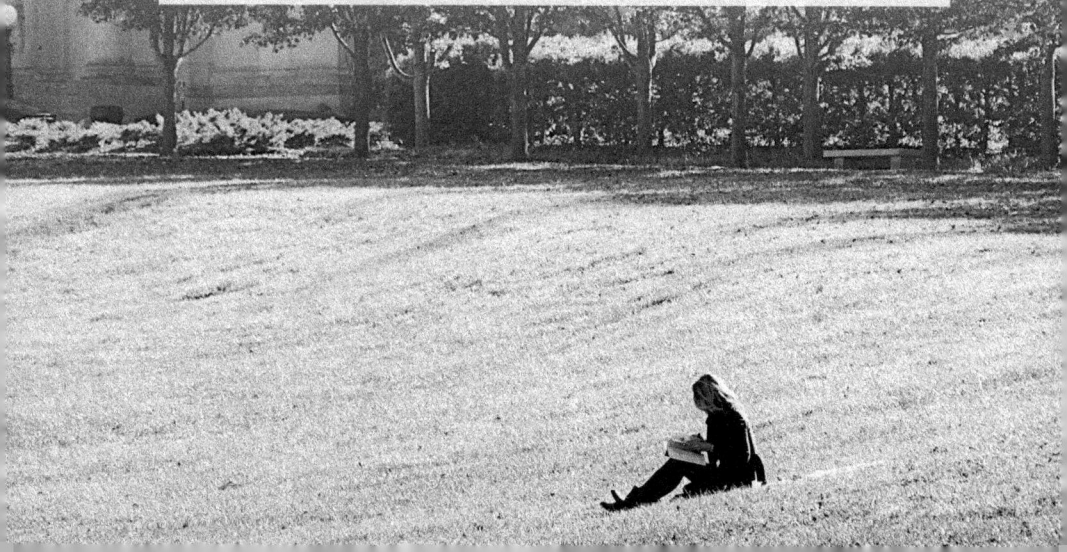

Simply Breathe: The Power of Presence

In Simply Breathe, we learn how mindfulness, being in the present moment, helps ease stress by calming our body and mind. We start noticing our present-moment experience by focusing on our breath as it's occurring. Since our breath occurs effortlessly, there's nothing we need to do but become aware of the breath as it flows in and out of our body. "Noticing" experience is the first skillset in my program because it is the foundation of all the other mindfulness skills. To become aware of the experience you are having, which is essential to all mindfulness-based skills, you must start noticing it.

📄 EXERCISE

Simply Breathe Exercise

Sit comfortably with your eyes open or closed. Take three deep breaths and see if you can notice where your breath is occurring most strongly in your body at this moment. It may be around your lips and nostrils, in the rise and fall of your belly, or the rise and fall of your chest. Next, see if you can follow it from inhalation to exhalation, and back again, or from fullness to emptiness. Do this for a few minutes. When thoughts, feelings, or sensations try to hijack your attention, note them and return your attention to your breath. You can also think to yourself, "Breathing in, I breathe in. Breathing out, I breathe out." Don't judge your experience but simply notice it. After a few moments, take three more deep breaths and open your eyes if they're closed.

Soothe Your Body: The Power of Paying Attention

In Soothe Your Body, we learn to direct our attention intentionally instead of letting it wander aimlessly. We deliberately tune in to the experiences in our body to retrain our minds to go where we want, unlike an "unruly puppy" (Ronald Siegel, PsyD, *The Mindfulness Solution*). We can reduce stress further by imagining ourselves breathing warmth and comfort into the tight places.

─────────────── 📄**EXERCISE** ───────────────

Soothe Your Body Exercise

Sit comfortably, where you won't be disturbed for the next five minutes, with your eyes open or closed. Take three deep breaths in and begin noticing a part of your body where you are experiencing some discomfort. Rather than labeling it bad or being judgmental about it, simply notice the qualities of how it feels. Is it warm or cool? Loose or tight? Soft or hard? Vibrating with energy or still? Once you become aware of what it feels like, if you want, imagine yourself breathing warmth and relaxation into this part of your body, softening and loosening any discomfort. Take three more deep breaths and open your eyes if they're closed.

Savor the Moment: The Power of Savoring Sensory Experience

Savoring the moment involves sensing the experience that we're having through all five senses: sight, sound, touch, taste, and smell. Current research in positive psychology indicates that savor-enhancing experiences can improve mood and decrease stress. Savoring can be done with activities that already occur in our daily lives by focusing our awareness on sensory experience.

—————————— 🗎 EXERCISE ——————————

Savor the Moment Exercise

Pick an activity you perform daily, such as brushing your teeth, taking a shower, or washing the dishes. Pay attention with all five senses to what you're doing. Be aware of the sights, sounds, tastes, smells, and touches that accompany it. For example, if you choose washing the dishes, be aware of seeing the soap bubbles, smelling the scent of the dish soap, hearing the water running, or touching the dishes or bubbles.

When thoughts or feelings try to steal your attention, simply note them and go back to focusing on the sensory experience of what you're doing. Practice savoring the same experience four to five times a week.

Settle Your Thoughts: The Power of Letting Go

In Settle Your Thoughts, we learn to note that thoughts are occurring and to let them pass without getting too attached to them. We witness how they come and go and are constantly changing from moment to moment. We consider the idea that thoughts are not facts but instead, passing mental events. Likewise, we practice not getting caught up in the stories we tell ourselves, instead realizing that we can't know with certainty what's going to happen until it does.

--- 📄 **EXERCISE** ---

Settle Your Thoughts Exercise

Sit comfortably with your eyes open or closed in a quiet place where you will be undisturbed for the next five minutes. Take in three deep breaths and notice how thoughts come and go, one after the next. Resist the urge to start telling yourself a story about your thoughts, and instead, picture them changing from moment to moment, like waves on an ocean, leaves flowing down a stream or clouds passing through the sky. Your thoughts are always changing, but you, as the witness of your experience are constant like the ocean, the stream, or the sky. Let thoughts come into your awareness, and then let them go once you notice them. Do this for five minutes. Then take three deep breaths and open your eyes if they're closed. Practice this daily for a week.

Self-Compassion Always

Self-Compassion Always involves accepting yourself fully, strengths and flaws, without self-criticism or self-judgment. Many people, especially caregivers, women, and people in the helping professions, are much more critical of themselves than they are anyone else. Rather than paying attention to what they're doing right and how much they're doing for others, they often dwell on the mistakes they've made or how they could be doing better. In this skill set, we learn to "befriend ourselves," and be kind to ourselves like we are to others we love.

--- 📄 **EXERCISE** ---

Self-Compassion Always Exercise

Sit comfortably with your eyes open or closed in a quiet place, where you can sit undisturbed for 5 to 10 minutes. Think about this past week and recall a time when you were self-critical or judgmental of something you did or thought. Next, imagine that one of your friends or loved ones had done something that caused them to be critical or judgmental of themselves. Think of what you'd probably say to them and then say these words to yourself. For example, "Everyone makes mistakes. Stop being so hard on yourself. Think about all the good things you've done." Once you can say something self-compassionate and accepting, repeat this a couple of times. Then take three deep breaths and open your eyes if they're closed. Practice this daily for a week.

To learn more about Dr. Sanford, or to order her book, *Stress Less, Live Better: 5 Simple Steps to Ease Anxiety, Worry, and Self-Criticism*, you can go to www.praeclaruspress.com. It is also available on Amazon in both print or Kindle editions.

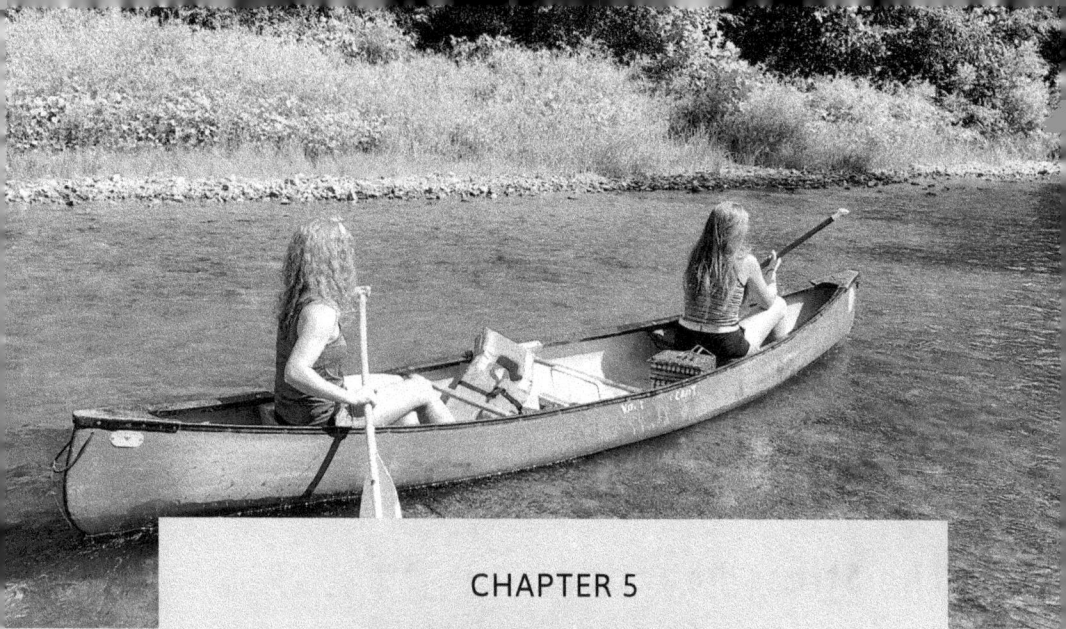

CHAPTER 5

SIMPLY BREATHE

The Power of Presence

When we are fully awake to the present moment, stress eases, and our body calms. This is mindfulness. Jon Kabat Zinn, who popularized this set of stress-reduction skills in the U.S., defined mindfulness as "Being aware of the present moment on purpose, without self-judgment." Unfortunately, research indicates that we don't spend much time in the present moment. Mindfulness skills can teach us how to re-inhabit the present moment and start to stress less and live better.

As human beings, we often create emotional suffering for ourselves by dwelling on worries about the future or regrets about the past. We get carried away with unpleasant thoughts, emotions, and bodily sensations. However, experience is always changing between negative, positive, and neutral aspects. By learning mindfulness skills, we can learn to cope in healthier ways and deal more skillfully with life's ups and downs.

Over the past 30 years, research has proven that mindfulness-based skills can reduce stress, depression, and anxiety, and improve our health and wellbeing. When practiced regularly, these skills, which have been around for thousands of years, have been effective in decreasing emotional suffering and pain and increasing joy and comfort.

The Stress Reaction

When we feel stress due to an imagined or actual threat, stress hormones, including adrenaline and cortisol, are released throughout our bodies as we prepare to fight or flee. Our inflammation levels increase. Our blood pressure and pulse rate accelerate. Blood gets directed to our limbs. Digestion decreases to enable us to use our energy more efficiently. Our pupils dilate, sharpening our ability to see a potential predator approaching us. Our senses become heightened. This stress reaction helped our ancient ancestors run and not get eaten by a saber-toothed tiger, ensuring the survival of our species.

Although human beings may have the most sophisticated brains of any species, our bodies and minds do not distinguish between external and internal threats, but react the same to both. This means that whether we are worried about our baby growing up to be a successful adult, or being hurt physically, our stress reaction will trigger. The more we pay attention to unpleasant thoughts, emotions, and bodily sensations, the stronger they become. The stories we tell ourselves about what's happened, or fears of what will occur, often make us feel unsettled.

Mind-body stress-reducing skills help us learn to direct our attention to where we want it to go instead of being pre-occupied with negative or unpleasant thoughts, emotions, and sensations.

Learning to direct our attention intentionally ultimately helps us learn to stress less and live better because we become able to choose which aspect of an experience we focus on. This doesn't mean we ignore negative thoughts, emotions, and sensations. It means we don't get carried away with them and create greater pain and suffering than we already have. Likewise, we begin to understand that all experience peaks and diminishes, and that even though a situation may seem unbearable at the time, this too shall pass.

Mindful or Mind Full?

Have you ever had the experience of driving in your car to get somewhere and you arrive at your destination 15 minutes later without noticing where you've been in between? I know I have and that this is a common occurrence. How does this happen? It's about paying attention. Most of us spend so much time thinking about thoughts that concern us, or telling ourselves stories about past events in our head. We miss what's happening in real-time. Our attention is elsewhere, and we need to learn to bring it back to the present moment to stress less and live better.

While all five mindfulness skillsets that I've compiled achieve this, we start in class with the Simply Breathe skillset because all it requires is noticing our present moment experience by noticing our breath. The wonderful thing about breathing is that we don't have to do anything for it to occur. Our bodies breathe spontaneously. To begin strengthening our mindfulness muscle, we notice the breath without trying to change it. The goal is not relaxation or finding nirvana. It is to have the simple experience of noticing our breath as it flows in and out of our body. That's it.

Many of my students wonder how something this simple can help them stress less and live better. Since the body doesn't distinguish between internal and external threat, the mental stress of worry, regret, unpleasant emotions, and negative thoughts activate the stress reaction like the physical threats our ancestors sought to avoid. In Buddhism, mindfulness helps quiet stress-triggering thoughts. Buddha, who it is said developed mindfulness to end human suffering, said this:

> When touched with a feeling of pain, the uninstructed person, sorrows, grieves, and laments beats his breast and becomes distraught. So, he feels two pains: physical and mental. Just as if they were to shoot a man with an arrow, and right afterward, were to shoot him with another one so that he would feel the pain of two arrows.

Like Buddha's students, we can learn mindfulness skills to stop feeding our fearful, anxiety-driven thoughts, feelings, and sensations, and instead acquire a more balanced and healthy perspective on our lives.

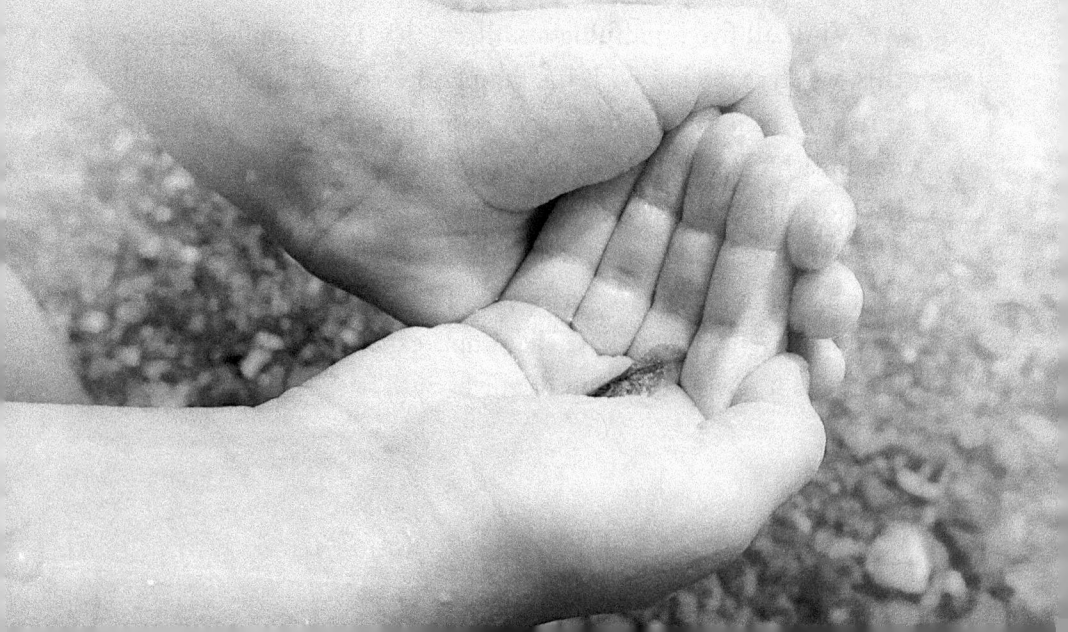

--------------------- 📄 **EXERCISE** ---------------------

Simply Breathe Exercise: Noticing the Breath

Before going further, let's practice the first breath exercise we do in my class. First, make certain you are in a comfortable and quiet setting where you can practice undisturbed for 5 to 10 minutes. Perhaps you have a place that feels restful and soothing to you, or you may want to create a place for yourself before starting. Having a comfortable chair, sofa, pillows, or blankets to cushion your body can be helpful. You may want to dim the lights or light a candle. If you are sitting on a mat on the floor, make certain your back is supported, so you aren't uncomfortable.

Remember, you are having a simple experience. You are not striving to feel relaxed or rid yourself of all thoughts. You will probably spend much of your time being distracted by thoughts, emotions, and sensations. This is normal and may vary depending on how you're feeling. Approach yourself with self-compassion like you would with a young child or friend. Whatever happens is fine. There is no right or wrong way to practice mindfulness. Each time you redirect your attention to your breath, you are easing stress and cultivating calm.

After you have a comfortable place where you can practice without interruptions for the next 10 minutes, either gently close your eyes or leave them open if this feels better to you. As you notice your breath, see if you can tell where you're experiencing it most in your body at this moment. It may be around your lips and nostrils, or in the rise and fall of your chest, or the rise and fall of your belly. Take a few moments to see if you can notice where it's occurring the strongest.

Once you've found where your breath is most noticeable, see if you can follow your breath from inhalation to exhalation and back again, or from fullness to emptiness and back again. When your attention wanders from your breath to a thought, emotion, or another sensation, gently and lovingly bring it back. Do not judge yourself or become self-critical by thinking, "I'm not doing this right," or "I must be the only one in the room who's having trouble with this." All of us have trouble with this, especially when we're starting to practice.

Spend a few minutes observing your breath and then release your attention on your breath and let it drift back to your physical presence in the room. Notice the chair, sofa, mat, or wall against which your body is seated. Notice sensations in your upper torso, lower torso, arms, legs, hands, feet, neck, shoulders, the front of your face, and the back of your head. You may want to move slowly or gently stretch, and if your eyes are closed, open them when you're ready. Sit quietly for a few moments and bring your attention to the experience you've just had.

✏️ Note-icing Your Experience

While sitting quietly, you may want to explore the following questions. If you like to keep a journal, this would be a good time to get it out and write down your answers to consider later.

* ✳ What bodily sensations did you notice?

* ✳ What did you notice about how you felt before the exercise and how you feel now? Were there changes you were aware of at different points in the exercise?

* ✳ If thoughts and emotions distracted you, what was it like to attempt to redirect your attention to your breath? Were there differences in how easy or difficult this was at different times?

✳ How could you take what you may have learned from this experience and use it to stress less and live better in your daily life?

Focused Breathing

The second skill in this skillset is called "focused breathing." Like the first exercise, we practice directing our attention intentionally rather than getting carried away with random thoughts, feelings, or sensations. To do so, we focus on a phrase or mantra as the object of our attention that is easier for some people than noticing the breath. One goal of the Stress Less, Live Better program is to learn many different skills to draw upon when you feel stressed. Each skill set is made up of several exercises so you can choose which one works best for you and practice that. I suggest you try each one.

Using a simple phrase paired with the in-breath and out-breath works better for some students than noticing the breath because it gives their overactive minds something to focus on. We often say, "In calm. Out stress," or "Breathe in. Breathe out." If you have a mantra, you can focus on that. Again, the goal is to have a simple experience, whatever happens, and practice directing our attention more intentionally.

─────────── 📄 EXERCISE ───────────

Simply Breathe: Focused Breathing

Now, let's practice the second exercise we do in class. First, make certain you are in a comfortable, quiet setting where you can practice undisturbed for 5 or 10 minutes. Perhaps you have a place that feels restful and soothing to you, or you may want to create a place for yourself before starting. Having a comfortable chair, sofa, pillows, or blankets to cushion your body can be helpful. You may want to dim the lights or light a candle. If you are sitting on the mat on the floor, make certain your back is supported so it isn't painful.

Remember, you are having a simple experience. You are not trying to feel relaxed or rid yourself of thoughts. You will probably spend much of your time being distracted by thoughts, emotions, and sensations. This is normal and may vary depending on the day and how you feel. Approach yourself with self-compassion like you would a young child or friend. Whatever happens is fine. There is no right or wrong way to practice mindfulness. Each time you redirect your attention to your breath, you are easing stress and cultivating calm.

After you have a comfortable place where you can practice without interruptions for the next 10 minutes, either gently close your eyes or leave them open if this feels better to you. Start noticing your breath and see if you can tell where you're experiencing it most in your body at this moment. It may be around your lips and nostrils, or in the rise and fall of your chest, or the rise and fall of your belly. Take a few moments to see if you can notice where it's occurring most strongly.

Once you've found where your breath is most noticeable, direct your attention to the phrase, "In calm. Out stress," or the "Breathe in. Breathe out." For a mantra, if saying something that has no specific meaning to you is easiest, I suggest you try *Om Bhavam Namah*. Loosely translated, this means "I am a field of infinite possibility," which is the essence of Deepak Chopra's First Spiritual Law. If you have training in Transcendental Meditation (TM) or Primordial Sound Meditation, you can use the mantra you were given. When you are distracted by thoughts, noises, or bodily sensations, gently and lovingly bring your attention back to your phrase or mantra. Do this for five minutes so you give yourself enough time for stress to begin to ease and your mind to settle. Whatever happens is fine.

After five minutes, release your phrase or mantra, and sit quietly and breathe. Direct your attention back to your physical presence in the room. Notice the chair, sofa, mat, or wall against which your body is seated. Notice sensations in your upper torso, your lower torso, your arms, your legs, your hands, your feet, your neck, your shoulders, the front of your face, and the back of your head. You may want to move slowly or gently stretch, and if your eyes are closed, open them when you're ready. Sit quietly for a few moments, paying attention to the experience you've just had.

✏️ *Note-icing Your Experience*

While sitting quietly, you may want to explore the following questions. If you like to keep a journal, this would be a good time to get it out and write down your answers to consider later.

- ✳ What bodily sensations did you notice?

- ✳ What did you notice about how you felt before the exercise and how you feel now? Were there changes you were aware of at different points in the exercise?

- ✳ If thoughts and emotions distracted you, what was it like to attempt to redirect your attention to your breath? Were there differences in how easy or difficult this was at different times?

- ✳ How could you take what you may have learned from this experience and use it to stress less and live better in your daily life?

Mindful-Minis for Simply Breathe: If You're Pressed for Time

Here are some suggestions for how to practice Simply Breathe when you're pressed for time.

* ❋ When you're at a stoplight, take three deep breaths in and out.

* ❋ If you're waiting in line at the grocery store, take five deep breaths in and out.

* ❋ While you're waiting in the carpool line, take five deep breaths.

* ❋ If you commute to work on a bus or metro line, take three deep breaths when you leave your residence and three when you return.

* ❋ Before you put your baby down in their crib, breathe in to the count of three and out to the count of three. Do this each time you pick them up.

* ❋ Before you get out of bed in the morning, breathe in to the count of three and out to the count of three for five times. Do this getting in at night too.

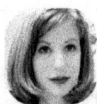

Megan's Mindful-ish Moment: Getting Started with Mindfulness Practice

When I started a formal mindfulness practice, I had the advantage of doing so in a group setting. Although some people feel too vulnerable lying prone with their eyes closed (you couldn't pay me to do the lying leg press at the gym), Diane did a good job creating a safe space. Most of the "mindful moms" in my class liked to do the exercises lying on their backs on yoga mats, eyes closed, sometimes with pillows underneath their heads or lower backs for comfort, and sometimes underneath a blanket. A few preferred to sit with their backs against a wall. Occasionally, for a change of pace, Diane would have us sit on cushions with legs crossed or practice walking meditation.

I say practicing in a group was an advantage because, as a beginner, I felt validated hearing about others' experiences and finding they often mirrored my own. Perhaps even more valuable than validation were the insights these other moms offered. For example, in one exercise you will read about in Chapter 8, Diane encouraged us to visualize our thoughts as clouds passing in the sky or whatever image worked best for us. In sharing the different images each of us chose, we provided each other with options we would not have thought of ourselves, some of which might work even better than the image we started with.

If your first exposure to mindfulness will involve practicing solo, I recommend that you read through the instructions for an exercise once or twice, then use the guided meditations at www.drdianesanford.com. Since you won't be getting outside validation from members of a group, make sure to remind yourself that getting distracted by thoughts, or having trouble with visualization, is completely normal and do not constitute failure. You wouldn't expect to become an amazing basketball player or concert pianist without practice; the same goes for mindfulness. But mindfulness does differ from the skills above in that, while there is a wrong or less-skilled way of playing a sport or instrument, there is neither a right nor a wrong way to practice mindfulness. If outside thoughts intrude as you try to follow your breath, that is a valid experience. Just bring your attention back to your breath and the present moment whenever you notice this happening. That's mindfulness practice—it can be as simple as that!

When I began to practice following my breath, I could usually do it for a few minutes, especially when Diane was speaking. After that, something would usually distract me. Occasionally, sounds from outside or the awareness of someone else following her breath beside me would break my concentration, but my thoughts were what sidetracked me the most. For many people, it is difficult to be silent and still without our minds starting to go squirrelly. We lead such busy lifestyles; it seems that in the rare moments we are not accomplishing something, we seek to be diverted by one of our electronic devices. In class, soon after Diane would stop directing us, my mind would start making lists, thinking about what I had to do next, worrying about what my daughter was doing, basically anything but what was happening at the moment. This is a habit many of us return to in the absence of other distractions. It can contribute to insomnia, keeps us from enjoying the present moment, and prevents us from taking time for necessary rest and renewal.

Despite setbacks, I kept practicing, and now simply breathing is the skill I find myself returning to most often in times of stress. Whenever I get stuck in traffic or frustrated at Luca for wasting time, I take a moment to follow my breath, and it calms me down, sometimes just a little and sometimes completely. Before I discovered mindfulness, the recommendation of taking a few deep breaths to calm down rarely worked for me. I needed that formal practice to learn how to use breath to reduce stress.

When practicing focused breathing, I use the Sanskrit mantra *Ohm Bhavam Namah*. I have found that using mantras with English words can become a slippery slope for me. If I silently repeat, for example, "In calm, out stress," I often make associations with those words until I eventually have complete and unrelated inner monologues. As you begin to practice focused breathing, try out different mantras until you find the one that works best for you.

At the risk of sounding trite, mindfulness is a journey, not a destination. Even once you have become more skilled at these exercises, it is critical to continue to practice. You may get derailed if you find yourself unusually busy. Don't beat yourself up over it; just resume your practice as soon as you can. Eventually, mindfulness can transition from a skill set to a mindset, as it did for me. Now I find that even when I'm not practicing formally or informally, knowing that my mindfulness skills are available to me is a comfort.

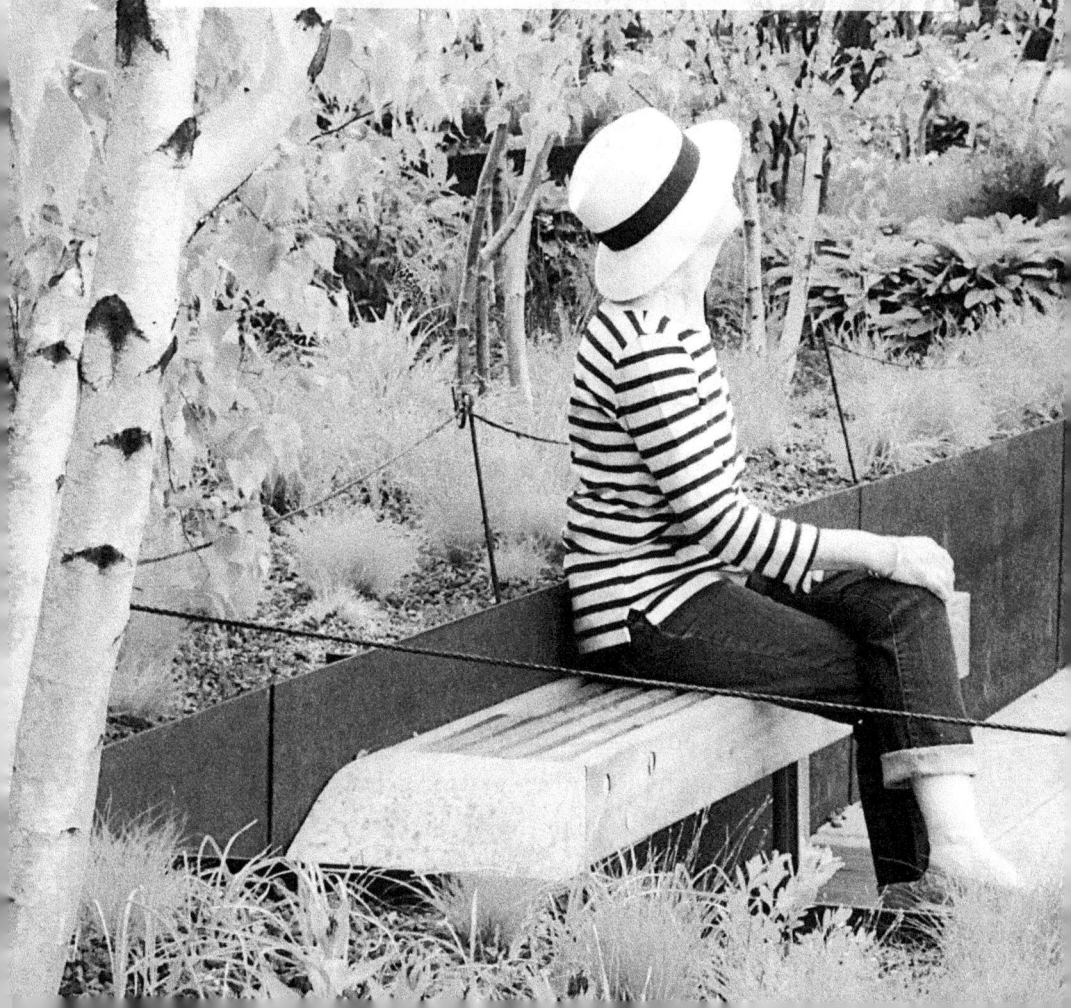

Creating Comfort

Like we mentioned earlier in this book, mindfulness-based skills need to be combined with self-care for optimal health and well-being for pregnant and postpartum moms. To improve your comfort, we suggest that you start by making your environment pleasing. Nourish your sense of smell with relaxing scents, like lavender or rose, freshly cut flowers, and candles you like. Nourish your sense of touch with comfy slippers, a fleecy robe, or a soft blanket. Nourish your sense of taste with soothing teas, healthy snacks, including fruit and veggies, and comfort food that's not too high in sugar or carbs.

Next, create a place you can go at the end of a long day or take a restful break. Decorate it with pictures and visuals that you like, and that help you unwind. Keep it tidy and uncluttered for maximum relaxation. Provide music, natural sounds, or white noise that is soothing. Many of us take time making certain our babies' rooms will be peaceful and calm for their comfort. Now, do it for yourself.

Motherhood and Presence

Most new moms find it difficult to direct their attention to the present moment because they focus on what's ahead and planning for it. They often get carried away with fearful thoughts about the future, even imagining their infants as teens and the trouble they may get into.

However, we need to equally consider that the present moment will not come again and it is here that we will find contentment and joy in our lives with our children and families. If we want our children to feel secure and safe in the world, they must know that we are here beside them with our full attention and love. Remember self-care is not a luxury; it is a necessity if we want to create healthy families and communities where our children and their children can flourish for generations yet to come.

CHAPTER 6

SOOTHE YOUR BODY

The Power of Paying Attention

In the last chapter, Simply Breathe, we learned to notice our moment to moment experience. In this chapter, we build on that skill by paying attention to different experiences in our bodies. This means that we learn to direct our attention intentionally and place it where we want it to go instead of letting it wander.

We say in class that as we progress from being less skillful to more skillful, we are still human and will make mistakes and get carried away. If we're having a day when we're tired and nothing is going right, we are likely to be more reactive and default to our less-skilled or autopilot reaction. Imagine that you're sitting in traffic after a long day and someone cuts you off. It would be normal to react in a stressful way, feeling angry and upset.

Now imagine that it's a beautiful day out, you've just finished a tasty meal, and you've spread out a blanket to take a nap. A car drives by with the radio blaring and stirs up some dust that scatters on your blanket, disturbing your rest. You feel annoyed and unsettled but quickly return to enjoying a calm and contented mood, despite the disruption. This is normal too.

The problem occurs when it's a beautiful day out, but our mind is so full of worry about the future or regrets about the past that we trigger our stress reaction without awareness or intention. The goal of mindfulness is to learn how to harness our attention so we can respond with choice rather than react on autopilot. By tuning into how our bodies feel in the moment, we can learn to do this. Body-centered awareness activities, like the ones in this chapter, give us tools to pay attention by focusing on raw experience and not our thoughts about it.

Unlike some of the traditional body-centered skills, the exercises in this chapter are also intended to cultivate a sense of relaxation and ease. Although we start by paying attention to how our bodies feel, we invite feelings of comfort and relaxation in as well. Because of this, I call the body-scan exercise I teach Body-Scan Relaxation instead of simply Body Scan, where we only observe what's happening without making any effort to change it. The reason for adding relaxation to the Body Scan is because many of us experience stress by tensing the muscles in our body. Paying attention to where we feel tension can help release it. Likewise, the intention of deliberately relaxing enables us to cultivate a state of greater ease and calm at the moment.

Pleasure and Pain

Experts in many disciplines, ranging from psychology to theology, agree that human beings tend to pursue pleasure and avoid pain, a seemingly wise choice. However, mindfulness programs teach that all experience is impermanent and constantly shifting between pleasant, neutral, and unpleasant thoughts, emotions, and bodily sensations. By pursuing pleasure and avoiding pain, we tend to hold onto negative experiences instead of allowing them to move through us and diminish in intensity.

Recall the metaphor of the Two Arrows, where the person who has not studied mindfulness feels two pains. The first is the arrow striking our skin. The second is the mental suffering created by dwelling on how bad it feels. If we pay attention to the raw experience we're having and explore the bodily sensations that occur, we may have less pain because our muscles are less likely to tighten and constrict, which increases pain. This also sounds counterintuitive. We think that by paying attention, we'll make things worse, but this belief is not true. Investigating how we feel with an open, non-judging mind can lessen pain and suffering.

Students in my classes frequently find that when they pay attention to the discomfort and tension in their bodies, their pain begins to ease. Instead of making things worse, pain and tightness diminish and they feel better. By facing what's happening, they allow themselves to experience their discomfort in a different, more manageable, and "skillful" way.

--------------------- 📄 EXERCISE ---------------------

5-Minute Tension Reliever

This is an exercise I teach in class and individual counseling sessions because it only takes 5 minutes. People often feel better just noticing where they're holding tension and not trying to make it go away. As with the exercises in Simply Breathe, find a spot where you can be undisturbed for the next 5 minutes. You can do this at your desk at work or in carpool line when you're waiting to pick up your children.

Gently and lovingly close your eyes and begin to pay attention to where you are experiencing tension in your body at this moment. For many people, it occurs in their neck and shoulders, or their chest or their bellies. Wherever you notice it, remember that you have a simple experience and that your experience is just that: your experience.

Whatever happens, do not judge yourself or become critical of what's occurring. Instead, notice your body tension as if exploring it for the first time. Note qualities of sensation rather than judging yourself for feeling pain or discomfort. For example, pay attention to sensations of warmth, coolness, vibration, lack of vibration, tightness, sharpness, flexibility, or rigidity. Be prepared for the sensations to vary as you pay attention. See what happens for you as you investigate this.

Notice the muscle tension for a minute or two, and then redirect your attention to the rise and fall of your breath at your belly. Experiment with intentionally directing your breath to the tight or tense places in your body, softening and loosening them with each inhalation, and letting go of stress and tension with each exhalation. Do this for a minute or two, not expecting anything to happen, just noticing what does.

Finally, imagine yourself breathing your whole body from the tip of your toes to the top of your head, softening and loosening all the muscles in your whole body. Imagine that you're becoming more spacious with each inhalation, and less tight and constricted with each exhalation. Do this for a minute. Then, redirect your attention back to your physical presence, noticing feelings in your upper torso, lower torso, arms, legs, hands, feet, neck, shoulders, the front of your face, and the back of your head. You may want to wiggle or gently stretch, and when you are ready, gently and lovingly open your eyes.

🖊 *Note-icing Your Experience*

While sitting quietly, you may want to explore the following questions. If you like to keep a journal, this would be a good time to get it out and write down your answers for later.

- ❋ What bodily sensations did you notice?

- ❋ What did you notice about how you felt before the exercise and how you feel now? Were there changes you were aware of during this exercise?

- ❋ If thoughts and emotions distracted you, what was it like to attempt to redirect your attention to your body? Were there differences in how easy or difficult it was to do this during this exercise?

- ❋ How could you take what you may have learned from this experience and use it to stress less and live better?

Pleasure, Pain, and Motherhood

Like most life experiences, motherhood is a mixed bag filled with positive and negative emotions, and pleasurable and painful moments. Anyone who tells you otherwise is lying. Motherhood can be blissful and despairing. We love our children more than we ever could have imagined, but we worry about them constantly and fear that some danger we haven't anticipated will threaten their health and wellbeing. We look at them in awe but then they start crying, peeing, pooping, and spitting up, and we feel physically drained and emotionally depleted. Motherhood is a psychological marathon, and it takes much emotional stamina and a lot of physical energy to stay in the race.

Motherhood is also an opportunity to practice mindfulness by coming to terms with the idea that we can't always expect our lives to be pleasant and stress-free. To be able to cope most skillfully with the changes new motherhood brings, we must learn to accept pleasure and pain without getting too carried away with either. We can learn to enjoy our babies even though we sometimes have negative feelings about them or being a mom. This is the nature of life. When we learn to accept motherhood as a mixed bag, we can ease stress and emotional suffering. For now, take my word for it and keep reading.

📄 EXERCISE

THE BODY-SCAN RELAXATION

Now, let's practice the body-scan relaxation. First, make certain you are in a comfortable, quiet setting where you can practice undisturbed for 15 minutes. In class, we do this exercise lying down on a yoga mat with pillows supporting our head and neck. Some students will lie flat, while others put a pillow under their knees for extra back support. Make certain you are in a position that feels comfortable to you, even if you adjust your posture during the exercise to ease discomfort. This is okay.

Close your eyes or keep them open if you want, and gently and lovingly take a few deep breaths. Next, notice where you are experiencing the breath most strongly in your body at this moment. It may be around your lips and nostrils, or in the rise and fall of your belly, or the rise and fall of your chest. Do not attempt to change it but see if you can follow it for a few breaths from inhalation to exhalation and back again, or from emptiness to fullness and back again.

Once you've followed your breath for a minute or two, direct your awareness to your feet and notice what your feet feel like.

Observe sensations of vibration or lack of vibration, tightness or looseness, warmth or coolness, or whatever you notice — experiment with not labeling them good or bad. You are having a simple experience, and there is no right or wrong way to participate in this exercise. Pay attention to the bodily sensations in your feet. Then use your calming breath to breathe relaxation and comfort into any of the tight places in your feet, softening and loosening them.

After your feet, move onto your knees, ankles, calves, and shins. Notice the sensations in these body parts. Notice how they feel. Are they tight or loose? Is there a sense of warmth or coolness, or vibration or lack of vibration? Do they feel flexible or rigid? For the next few moments, experience what it feels like in your knees, ankles, calves, and shins. Then if you like, take your calming breath to breathe relaxation and comfort into any of the tight places, softening and loosening them.

Next, focus your attention on your upper legs, muscles and joints in your upper leg and hip socket. Repeat the same steps as you did for your feet and your lower legs. Once you notice the sensations in this part of your body for a few moments, use your calming breath to breathe relaxation and comfort into any of the tight places, softening and loosening them.

One at a time, move on to your lower torso-abdomen, buttocks, colon, intestines, and genitals; followed by your upper torso-stomach, diaphragm, lungs, heart, and kidneys; followed by all the parts of your upper arms, then your lower arms, then your wrist, palm, and fingers.

Next, notice what your neck and shoulders feel like; the front of your face and the back of your head. Finally, scan your whole body for any remaining tension and discomfort, breathing warmth and relaxation into anywhere that's needed.

If you fall asleep during this exercise, it means that you're tired and require rest. Don't judge or criticize yourself for this. Many of my students, from postpartum moms to women having sleep disturbances brought on by menopause, use this exercise to help them fall asleep. It is one of the best remedies I know for insomnia or waking during the night and not being able to turn your brain off to fall back to sleep.

There are many versions of the body scan with and without relaxation. The easiest way to learn the body-scan relaxation I teach in class, and have summarized for you above, is to listen to the download available at www.drdianesanford.com. It's often easier when you're learning these skills to have audio to guide you, so you don't get stressed out trying to remember what comes next. As always, see what works best for you.

✏️ Note-icing Your Experience

While sitting quietly, you may want to explore the following questions. If you like to keep a journal, this would be a good time to get it out and write down your answers to look at later.

* What bodily sensations did you notice?

* What did you notice about how you felt before the exercise and how you feel now? Were there changes you were aware of at different points in the exercise?

* If thoughts and emotions distracted you, what was it like to attempt to redirect your attention to your body? Were there differences in how easy or difficult it was to do this during this exercise?

* How could you take what you may have learned from this experience and use it to stress less and live better in your life?

Body Wisdom

Our bodies can help inform us about how we are experiencing life if we choose to listen. Unlike our minds, which are constantly telling us stories about how life is, the body is more likely to inform us in a raw, uncensored way about how experience is affecting us.

For example, consider the experience of grief. When a loved one dies, the grieving person has trouble eating, consumes less food, and eats less often. They may have a pit in their stomach or a feeling of emptiness. Their sleep is disturbed, and they have trouble falling and staying asleep. Their surroundings seem unreal and foreign. They may feel numb and detached from other people. Some can't stop crying while others feel a physical ache in their heart and bones. The life they've known is gone, and they are confronted with many bodily sensations that mirror what's happening in their emotional lives. Those of us who have lost a loved one know how much our bodies physically experienced the loss as we struggled to adjust mentally and emotionally.

When we fall in love, our bodies let us know that something is different. Like grief, we may have trouble eating or sleeping. Our hearts feel full, bursting with joy. We get excited to see our loved one and feel butterflies in our stomachs. We may be distracted and pay less attention to what's going on around us. We feel giddy, light-headed, and often can't stop smiling. Our senses are sharp and vibrating with energy. We are filled with pleasant thoughts, emotions, and bodily sensations.

Whether we are grieving or falling in love, the sympathetic nervous system activates our bodies in similar ways, which is why we may have trouble distinguishing excitement from stress. Butterflies in our stomach can signal either unpleasant or pleasant emotion. Next, let's see what happens when our body wisdom short circuits or we don't listen to it.

Body Wisdom and Addictive Behaviors

Because most of us are convinced that seeking pleasure and avoiding pain is the way to live, we are unprepared to skillfully weather life's ups and downs. We are certain that if we let the pain surface, it will not go away and we will be unhappy for a long time. The opposite is true. As we learn to be present in the experience we are having, we discover that the intensity of our pain peaks and diminishes over time. The problem is clinging to pleasant sensations and ignoring or avoiding the unpleasant ones. Addictive behaviors often develop as a less skillful way of coping with stress and pain.

Let's turn first to our addiction to food that has become an epidemic in U.S. culture. Current research indicates that one-third of the U.S. population has a BMI >30, another one-third has a BMI 26-29, and the remaining one-third is average weight. What does this have to do with paying attention to body wisdom? Body wisdom is a significant factor in our addiction to food and can help us learn more skillful ways of dealing with stress.

Part of the problem is that we are not aware of our bodies much of the time. We don't pay attention or ignore our body's signals that we are hungry, tired, or stressed. We often eat in our cars or in front of the television, or we have our cellphones on and may be texting or reading something online. We eat quickly so we can get to what's next, not noticing when we start to feel full or savoring what we are eating.

Because we spend so much time living in our heads and outside our bodies, we miss the opportunity for eating to be emotionally satisfying and nourishing. Likewise, we consume food or indulge in our food cravings to avoid an unpleasant experience. Stress increases and before we know it, we're eating a container of ice cream, or a bag of M&Ms, with little awareness of what's going on emotionally.

All we know is that we want to escape the unpleasant feelings or bodily sensations we're experiencing, and food numbs us out or quiets our mounting dis-ease. However, the fix is only temporary, so to keep the unpleasant feelings and sensations from resurfacing, we overeat or make poor choices. Although food addiction is a less-skillful way of coping, it keeps us from facing what's troubling us.

Alcohol, drugs, work, compulsive exercise, sex addiction, addiction to video games, or addiction to social media are other less-skillful ways of avoiding or ignoring our emotional lives. In the moment, these addictions or compulsions alleviate stress and pain, but over time, lead to emotional distress and physical discomfort.

Cultivating more skillful ways to weather life's ups and downs, like the ones described in this book, takes more effort, self-discipline, ongoing commitment, persistence, and the willingness to face the things that scare us. Yet, it is a more effective long-term solution.

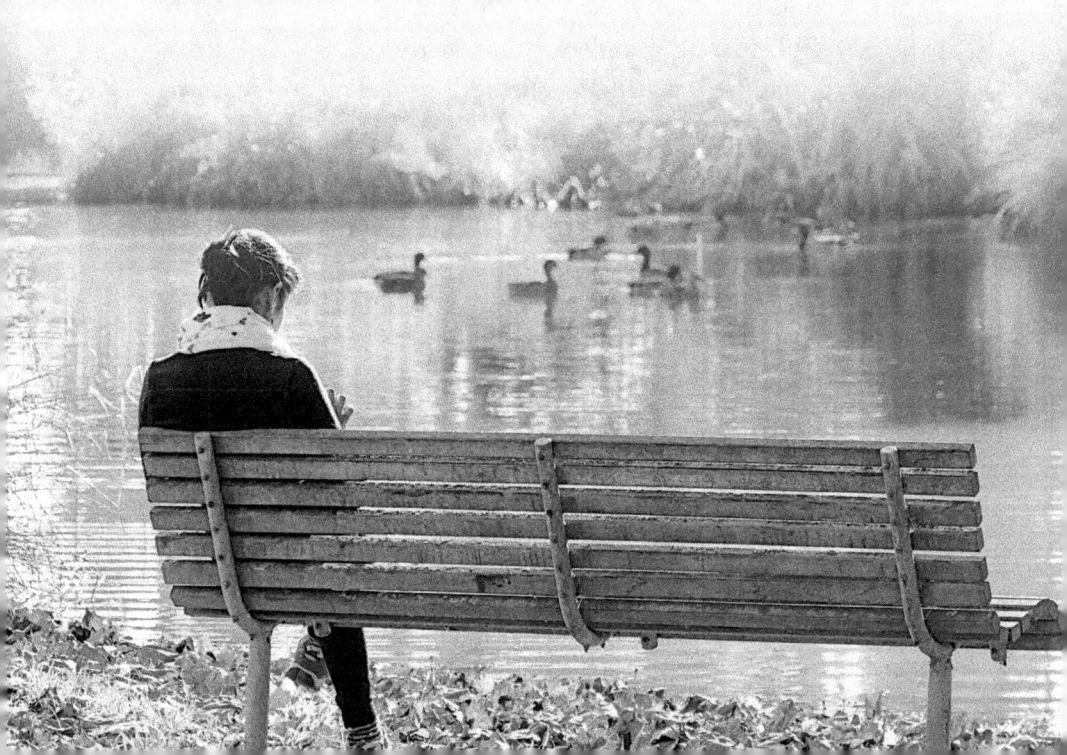

Learning to Pay Attention to Your Body's Wisdom

The exercises introduced in this skillset, Soothe Your Body, help us learn to listen to our body's inner wisdom. We focus on how our bodies feel, whether our sensations are pleasant, neutral, or unpleasant. We begin to resist the urge to turn away from unpleasant sensations. Instead, we investigate the qualities of our bodily sensations and learn to pay attention to what is occurring.

As we start to pay attention to what's happening in our bodies rather than labeling it pleasant or unpleasant, we may discover that tension or discomfort begins to ease. By dealing with pleasant, neutral, and unpleasant bodily sensation, we increase our capacity to cope with unpleasant thoughts and feelings rather than ignore or push them away.

We begin strengthening our mindfulness muscle, which enables us to stress less and live better with whatever life change we are facing. Because of the physical changes that are part of pregnancy, postpartum, and early motherhood, we have many chances to practice listening to our body's wisdom and learning from it if we decide to.

Mindful-Minis for Soothe Your Body: If You're Pressed for Time

Here are some suggestions for how to practice Soothe Your Body when you're pressed for time.

* Give yourself a gentle neck or shoulder rub. Many people carry tension in their bodies here.

* When you're walking, slow your pace down and notice how your heels lift and lower as you move. Take 10 slow steps and count to three with each step.

❋ Curl and uncurl your fingers one at a time, starting with the right and then left hand. Do it five times on each hand.

❋ After you shower or bathe, massage lotion over your entire body from head to toe. Take three or more minutes for this.

❋ Lie down on a sofa or your bed, and notice different parts of your body sinking into the mattress. Start with your left ankle, then your torso, your chest, your right wrist, your left wrist, neck and shoulders, and head.

❋ Yoga is one of my favorite practices for mindful movement. You do not need to be a yoga pro to do the first two poses. If you have an interest in doing more, purchase Sara Ivanhoe's gentle yoga video, Candlelight Yoga. Practice the yoga poses below to get started.

Pose One: Corpse Pose, Final Relaxation or Savasanna

Lie down on your yoga mat or put a towel on the floor and let your arms and legs spread out comfortably. Remain in this position for 5 minutes, noticing how your belly rises and falls when you breathe.

Pose Two: Cat and Cow

Get down on your hands and knees, and make certain that your hands are aligned with your shoulders and there is a straight line between your knees and buttocks. Start by stretching your neck, shoulders, and back forward, and head up like a cat that's stretching. Then, round your back towards the ceiling and try to touch your nose to your belly button, like a cow. Repeat this entire sequence five times.

Pose Three: Child's Pose

Child's pose, if you are familiar with yoga, is a restorative pose that allows you to soothe your body and cultivate relaxation. Spend five minutes in child's pose but adjust your body or come out of the pose as needed. Always practice at your own pace and do as much as you can.

Motherhood and Paying Attention

Pregnancy and postpartum changes our bodies, which makes it impossible for us to ignore them. At the start of pregnancy, our breasts grow and swell, and we feel nausea and fatigue like nothing we've known. The miracle of our baby growing inside us is accompanied by profound physical changes, and many women suffer body-image issues during this time, as Megan will discuss later in this chapter. Likewise, they report differences in sexual desire with some becoming more interested in sex and others less.

By the second trimester, weight gain and symptoms of fluid retention start to become noticeable. We consume more food than we normally would to nourish ourselves and our growing baby. Many of us have rarely enjoyed food as much as we do then. When I asked my OB if gaining 9 pounds in one month was a problem, he told me only if I continued to do that for the remaining four months. We start to feel our baby moving, and while it often feels like gas at first, by the end of this trimester, it is steady and forceful, particularly when we lie down to rest.

The third trimester also brings many shifts in our body, preparing us for birth and breastfeeding. Oxytocin, the attachment hormone, increases to assist our progress towards labor and delivery and to ensure that we feel more biologically inclined to care for our infants. One byproduct of oxytocin is becoming highly attuned to others so that we notice the baby's discomfort and will do something to about it. When our baby cries or signals distress is some way, we automatically get uncomfortable. This biochemical change was designed to make certain that we protected our babies, so our species survived.

Within 24 hours after delivering the placenta, our progesterone and estrogen levels plummet to pre-pregnancy levels, further disrupting our endocrine and brain chemistry. Again, these hormone-related changes intensify any existing tendencies we have toward anxiety or depression because our brain chemistry is affected. While all women will experience the "baby blues," others will experience a clinical episode of anxiety and depression, and a much smaller number will experience postpartum psychosis. Reread Chapter 3 for guidelines on noticing changes that indicate anxiety or depression, and when to seek professional help.

The Pitfalls of Biologically Programmed Attention

Although these biologically programmed changes in our hormones were designed to make it more likely that we would protect our infants from harm, they often intensify the likelihood of us being unable to control our reactivity to unpleasant thoughts, feelings, and sensations. During early motherhood, when our hormones change, it is easier to get carried away with feelings and thoughts of an impending threat than before we birth our babies. This heightens our tendency to pay attention to cues from our infants and others, and situations that normally we would let go.

For example, most of the time when our babies cry, they are not in extreme distress or at risk of being harmed. But once our fight-flight alarm system is triggered, it's difficult for us to keep this in perspective like we normally could. Instead, we create alarming stories and overwhelmingly negative thoughts about peril coming to them. Although this is a challenging time to separate our fears of imagined threat from actual ones, mindfulness skills can keep us on track, despite feeling uneasy or alarmed. The more skillful we become, the more we can intentionally override our heightened distress reactions and calmly attend to our infant's needs without getting ourselves worked up and stressed out. In Chapter 7, we'll learn more ways to redirect our attention so this is less likely to occur, and we are more likely to learn to stress less and live better in early motherhood and beyond.

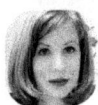

Megan's Mindful-ish Moment: Diets and Body Image Postpartum

Increasing mind-body awareness includes becoming aware of and questioning one's body *image*. Many of us celebrate the changes that occur in our bodies while we are pregnant because we are excited about the life growing inside of us. But how do we feel about the changes pregnancy has wrought when we're no longer pregnant? Remember what Diane said about the drastic drop in our hormone levels after we've delivered? Our excitement about our bodies and our self-esteem can drop just as drastically at approximately the same time.

While we are trying to conceive, pregnant, and postpartum, many of us will change our diet and lifestyle habits. Women who have tried and failed to quit smoking will suddenly stop, cold turkey, because they know the risks smoking poses to their unborn babies. Those of us who are accustomed to sipping on caffeinated beverages all day will have to drastically cut back on the coffee, switch to decaf, or find alternative ways of energizing. Some of us start watching our diets more carefully, focusing more on nutrient-dense whole foods rather than consuming empty calories. Others figure they're "eating for two" and allow themselves to indulge in treats they were never able to eat before without feeling guilty. For many of us, it's some combination of the two. We take our prenatal vitamins and avoid alcohol, sushi, raw cheeses, and the like. If we didn't before, we might start exercising more regularly (not too strenuously, of course). For some of us, prenatal yoga will be our first experience with both yoga and meditation.

Some of us may mistreat our bodies, whether it be through inadequate nutrition or overeating, poor sleep habits, substance abuse, or some other way. We may reason that it's okay because we're only hurting ourselves, although this is usually not the case. However we felt before getting pregnant, once we do, many of us can and will change our habits as we realize our bad choices will directly impact someone else—in the case of pregnancy, a fetus that is incapable of making its own choices.

But what happens after we deliver? I am picturing a poignant family tableau: me with a sleeping Luca's head cradled in one hand, a breast pump in the other, and Dave holding a slice of pizza to my mouth as I attack it like a feral dog. I think most new moms will find themselves in these types of situations. For the first few weeks and possibly months after your baby is born, you will count yourself lucky to get something edible in your mouth, never mind what it is. Eventually, though, many of us will start thinking about instituting a different way of eating.

So, at the risk of digressing, and before we talk about postpartum body image, let's talk about diets for a moment – and only a moment, because if you'd wanted to read a diet book, you would have chosen one among the 3.7 zillion available. You can trust me regarding the ubiquity of diet books (if not the exact figure) because I've read, to put it mildly, my fair share. I've also tried a number of these diets myself. There was a point in time when I was like the *Consumer Reports* of popular diets, so much so that my mother worried that I had an unhealthy preoccupation with food. My dad said, "Oh, leave her alone, JaJuan. It's her *hobby*."

I would call myself a nutritionist *manqué*, except for the fact that I tend to read the science-y stuff, decide whether it's plausible or not, and then promptly forget it. This can prove problematic when someone asks, "Why can't you eat that?" because I'll inevitably reply with something stupid like, "Uh… leptin resistance?" without knowing exactly what that is.

While I haven't retained everything I've read, it's still safe to say that I could fill a considerable-sized book (maybe one of the later *Harry Potters*) with what I know about dieting. One thing my research and personal experience has taught me can be summed up with a quote from *Bridget Jones's Diary*:

> I realize it has become too easy to find a diet to fit
> in with whatever you happen to feel like eating and
> that diets are not there to be picked and mixed but
> picked and stuck to, which is exactly what I shall
> begin to do once I've eaten this chocolate croissant.

Familiarity with a multitude of diets can cause trouble when you start "maintenance" and are making your own decisions. The thought process can go something like this: "Well, potatoes are okay on the Whole 30, cheese is kosher on South Beach, bacon is a staple of Atkins, butter is highly encouraged on the Wild Diet, and green onions are a vegetable! So sure, I'll take that loaded baked potato!" Most diets do agree on a few things – sugar is bad, green vegetables are good, and exercise helps. And that's where the similarities end,

I'm afraid.

Another thing I've learned is that most diet designers won't admit that their plans are, in fact, diets; rather, they're *lifestyles*. They will claim that diets don't work, the implication being that their approaches do because they're not diets. The claim that diets don't work is patently untrue. Conservatively, I would estimate that 95% of diets do work, if you follow them. The problem is that few of us have the willpower to follow a diet to the letter, and even fewer of us are willing to change our lifestyles forever. I can tell you from experience that the Atkins diet, for instance, does work for a time. I went on it many years ago near the beginning of the low-carb craze. I lost a considerable amount of weight in a very short amount of time. And three weeks in, I would have gouged out someone's eyes for a bowl of plain oatmeal.

The third and final thing I want to say about diets is probably the most important. Love yourself now, just as you are. You can go on a neverending quest for physical self-improvement, but no diet, exercise regimen, or cosmetic procedure in the world will give you self-esteem if you start with none. A critical part of mindfulness is living in the moment, and that means not dwelling upon some indeterminate future in which you weigh 10 or 100 pounds less, or next Monday, when you swear you will start working out again. The person you are right now is worthy of self-love and self-care. No, we should not be unhealthy and eat, drink, or smoke whatever we want all the time. Barring incredible medical advances with questionable ethics, the body you've got is the only one you're going to get in this life, so you should treat it with respect. Part of that is eating healthfully, exercising, and getting enough sleep, yes. But another part is accepting, and maybe even appreciating, your imperfections.

Let me give you an example from my own life. I was one of

those women who, despite all warnings to the contrary, was convinced that pregnancy would not change my body whatsoever. I imagined that my nine-months-pregnant self would look exactly like my pre-pregnancy self with a cute basketball-sized bump under my shirt, and I would bounce back like Heidi Klum and be ready for a Victoria's Secret fashion show six weeks afterward. Cue the laugh track.

First, it became clear to me that my pregnancy body was going to have completely different dimensions than expected because of how much water I was retaining. Yes, my belly got bigger, but so did my knees, my ankles, my arms, my face, and pretty much everything else. Second, after I gave birth, I still looked about four months pregnant. And did I bounce back after six weeks? Not even close. When Luca was 11 weeks old, we went to visit my sister-in-law and her family. I could finally wear my non-maternity, pre-pregnancy jeans and was feeling pretty good about myself. That is until my four-year-old nephew pointed to my midsection and said, "Aunt Megan, your belly's still big. I think you have another baby in there!" Kids say the darnedest things.

Still, I felt proud that, due to genetics or the diligent application of cocoa butter or both, I had gotten through pregnancy unscathed by stretch marks. My stomach, though rather squashier than before, remained perfectly unblemished. Then one day, about a month after Luca was born, I was engaged in the rare activity of styling my hair. Most of my clothes were still uncomfortable at that time, so I was delaying getting dressed for as long as possible. I turned away from the bathroom mirror, looked into a hand mirror to check the back of my hair, and realized with horror that I had somehow spent the previous ten months completely oblivious to my butt. It looked as if an entire colony of stretch marks had taken up residence there.

My first response was anger at my husband for never notifying me of this development. My second response was the urge to continue ignoring my butt for the next 10 months, or possibly the rest of my life. I didn't want to face the stretch marks, but it wasn't just that. Many other parts of my body had become objectionable to me as well.

When we moms compare our current bodies to what they were like before kids, we can feel pretty dejected. Maybe our hips are permanently wider or our stomachs more Rubenesque. Perhaps our breasts have migrated an inch or two south of where they previously resided. Even if we remain childless, our bodies will eventually change. We will lose muscle tone and the ability to "drop it low." We will get wrinkles and gray hairs. We have internalized the voice of our youth-obsessed society that says these things aren't beautiful. But we have to ask ourselves, who makes these rules? Is it the cosmetic surgeons who profit from facelifts and liposuction and vaginoplasty? Is it Hollywood with their seemingly endless supply of young starlets? Is it the modeling industry, the cosmetics industry, the fitness industry, the makers of Spanx? Or is it whatever misogynists propagated the idea that women's value lies in our sex appeal, so when that fades, we essentially have no value?

Don't get me wrong, I love makeup and clothes, and God bless the makers of Spanx. But as women, I do think it's important to question the source of our collective low self-esteem. If my Gender Studies background has taught me anything about that, it's to follow the money. When we do, it becomes abundantly clear that the rule-makers have some serious ulterior motives.

Eventually, armed with this thought, I went back to the mirror, took my clothes off, and looked at my body again. I endeavored not to judge or compare or evaluate, but to witness. And yes, the reflection did bear some of the signs some of my friends had warned me about when they said, "Pregnancy will wreck your body." But my body wasn't wrecked. It was healthy and strong and real. I had endured some pretty crazy and amazing things; I just had a few "battle scars" to prove it. My body wasn't perfect, but it reflected who I had become inside: someone who sacrificed a bit of her vanity for someone else, to bring another life into the world.

After I finished writing this, I asked my husband, "Why didn't you tell me when I started getting stretch marks on my butt?" He replied, "You have stretch marks on your butt?" Let me go on record and say that I am not a lights-off, get-out-of-bed-wearing-the-comforter type of individual. So take heart, my fellow warriors. While you're struggling to discover your inner and outer beauty, there are plenty of people who will find you beautiful in the meantime. Or maybe love really is blind.

CHAPTER 7

SAVOR THE MOMENT

The Power of Savoring

I n the previous chapter, we learned to pay attention to the experience of our bodily sensations from moment to moment. This chapter builds on that by extending our paying attention to bodily sensation to awareness of how experience affects all five senses: sight, touch, sound, smell, and taste. Current research in positive psychology indicates that savoring–enhancing strategies may increase overall life satisfaction and happiness (Bryant, Fred, & Veroff, 2007),

In a recent study of 300 participants (Quoidbach, Berry, Hansenne, & Nikolajck, 2010), investigators found that those who focused their attention on the present moment reported greater life satisfaction than those who were distracted. Likewise, they found that paying attention to the positive details rather than negative details of momentary experience resulted in more happiness and life satisfaction. The researchers concluded that people might need to cultivate multiple "savoring" strategies to achieve lasting happiness. The goal of this chapter is to introduce you to some of these skills.

Unlike other skill sets, "savoring" is directed towards a positive or neutral experience. Although mindfulness skills teach us to cope more skillfully with pleasant, neutral, and unpleasant bodily sensations, thoughts, and feelings, savoring is not practiced with an unpleasant experience. We deliberately choose *not* to focus on the negative aspects of what's occurring in our lives, so we don't trigger unpleasant bodily sensations, thoughts, and feelings. Like other mindfulness skills, savoring our experience strengthens our practice of directing our attention intentionally.

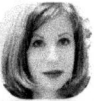

Megan's Mindful-ish Moment: The Myth of Multitasking

One big obstacle in achieving mindfulness is the attempt to multitask. When we become parents, multitasking takes on a whole new meaning. To some extent, it will be unavoidable – whatever we are doing, some part of our minds will always be on our child. Nevertheless, we should acknowledge the limits of multitasking and the value of savoring the present moment.

To live in the moment, we must be fully present, and we cannot be fully present if we are trying to do multiple things at once. In his book, *The Myth of Multitasking: How 'Doing it All' Gets Nothing Done,* business efficiency guru Dave Crenshaw puts forth a controversial argument, that so-called "multitasking" is less efficient than doing one thing at a time. This isn't just one person's theory; there is a substantial amount of research to back it up.

To begin, let's take a look at the origin of the term multitasking. As words go, this is a relatively new one. When it was first coined, it referred to a computer's apparent capacity to carry out multiple tasks simultaneously. Let me reiterate: it was something computers—not people—were doing. And as it turns out, even computers can't multitask; they can only switch between programs so quickly that it appears simultaneous.

The same thing is true for us. When we believe we are multitasking, we are doing what Crenshaw calls "switch-tasking," which is exactly what it sounds like. We are switching back and forth between tasks. Unfortunately, people aren't nearly as good at switch-tasking as computers are. Every time we switch tasks, our minds need to undergo a shift. Some of you are probably thinking, "Megan, you are so wrong, I can take a phone call and answer an email at the same time." I am sure we are all very accomplished individuals, each in our way, but the human brain doesn't work that way. The shift your mind undergoes between tasks may be near imperceptible to you, but it is still occurring, and it still costs you time

I'm not trying to suggest we stop switch-tasking altogether. A lot of times, we have no choice! I want us to realize what is going on when we think we are multitasking and what its limitations are. For instance, I frequently cook dinner and supervise Luca at the same time. I can get reasonably edible food on the table and make sure my daughter doesn't critically injure herself. That's about all I can expect from myself under the circumstances. I'm never going to become a top chef putting in less than my full attention and effort. And I'm not spending quality time with Luca with one eye on the stove and one hand on the wooden spoon.

That's okay with me. I don't aspire to be a top chef, and I still have plenty of time for teachable moments with my child. The problem comes in when one task does require our full and vigilant attention. I would suggest that multitasking is even more problematic because we can have trouble determining which task deserves the most attention, and to what degree. For example, during my ill-fated year of law school, I was convinced that I could play the computer game TextTwist and pay attention to the professor's lecture in Contracts class simultaneously. I could see enough of my fellow students' laptop screens to know I wasn't alone in my belief of being an excellent multitasker. I knew that learning Contracts took precedence over a computer game, so I should have allotted the most concentration to my professor. But unless I was doing recitation, TextTwist demanded the most immediate attention, being a time-sensitive endeavor, and thus, was given more importance than it warranted. Unfortunately, I was so immersed in the multitasking culture that I did not realize just how much I wasn't learning until I took my final exams.

In addition to its ability to derail our academic and professional endeavors, multitasking can be damaging to our interpersonal relationships. When we talk to our friends and family without giving them our full attention, it makes them feel as though they are unimportant to us, which is (hopefully) not the message we want to send. I admit that occasionally when someone is speaking to me, I am too busy thinking about what clever thing I can say next to give them my full attention. I would wager that most people would prefer a friend who is a good listener to one who is witty and articulate all the time.

Some of us are also guilty of checking our smartphones constantly, which is becoming more and more culturally acceptable but is a particularly blatant way of telling someone, "I am not giving you my full attention." Still, others of us have to be constantly moving and accomplishing something, which may make our companion believe that, for instance, having a freshly vacuumed floor is more important than what she has to say.

When we multitask, we tend to increase tension and discomfort. By intentionally choosing to "savor" our experience, we can experience greater ease and less stress. Again, this may seem counterintuitive to the idea of getting as much done in as short a time as possible, and that the longer things take to get done, the less efficient we are. So, let's look at this by exploring a common activity, eating, during which we frequently multitask. Then, you decide whether multitasking or savoring works best.

―――――――――― 📄 EXERCISE ――――――――――

Everyone's Favorite Mindful Chocolate Exercise

In traditional mindfulness practice, we first experience savoring or paying attention to our five senses by eating a single raisin. In my class, we start with a piece of chocolate, and of course, you get your choice of light or dark. If you're not a fan of chocolate, you may use whatever food you have that is small and bite-sized. The point is not what you choose, but how you approach this exercise. Again, the emphasis is on experiencing whatever you notice slowly through all five senses: sight, touch, sound, smell, and taste.

Begin by sitting comfortably on a chair, sofa, yoga mat, or cushion, where you can practice undistracted for the next 10 minutes. Take a few deep breaths and then place the chocolate or your bite-sized morsel in your hand. Look at the wrapped chocolate and see what you can discover about it as you roll it around in your palm. Is it shiny or dull? Is it grooved or smooth? Notice the qualities you perceive through your eyes. Then take the chocolate while it's still wrapped and put it between your thumb and middle finger and roll it around, paying attention to the sensation of touch. Is it rough or slick? Rigid? Pliable? Pay attention to what you discover through touch as you explore it.

Next, hold the chocolate up to your ear and see if you perceive any qualities of sound. This is usually when the class starts laughing and thinking this is silly. However, paying attention to the absence or presence of sound is another way of sharpening our awareness of sensory experience. Then, unwrap the chocolate and hold it under your nostrils. What do you smell? Is it fragrant or not? Sweet or spicy? Strong or weakly scented? Let your nose inform you about it.

After you've smelled the chocolate, put it in your mouth and let it rest on your tongue. Notice what happens inside your mouth. Do you start to salivate? What is it like to let it sit on your tongue without eating it? Slowly take a bite and experience the taste of the chocolate. Students often report more flavor than they've noticed before. Many report that they didn't know a single piece of chocolate could have tasted so good. Some mention that eating it mindfully made the experience more satisfying. When we savor our experience instead of racing through it, we notice how things seem different than what we've been conditioned to expect.

Finally, chew the piece of chocolate, let it dissolve and swallow. Once you've swallowed the whole piece, sit quietly and take mental note of what occurred. Focus on your awareness of the chocolate through all five senses: sight, touch, sound, smell, and taste.

✏️ Note-icing Your Experience

While sitting quietly, you may want to explore the following questions. If you like to keep a journal, this would be a good time to write down your answers to think about later.

❋ What did you notice about your sensory experience?

❋ What did you notice about how you felt before the exercise and how you feel now? Were there changes you were aware at different points in the exercise?

❋ If thoughts and emotions distracted you, what was it like to attempt to redirect your attention to your senses? Were there differences in how easy or difficult it was to do this during this exercise?

❋ How do you think this exercise is about savoring life more?

❋ How could you take what you may have learned from this experience and use it to stress less and live better?

--------------------- 🗎 EXERCISE ---------------------

Savoring What You're Doing Exercise

One of the things my clients love about this exercise is that you practice it with activities that are already part of your daily or weekly routine. The focus is to bring your full attention to the moment you're in and experience it with full sensory awareness. For example, when you're taking a shower, notice what's happening with your five senses. Pay attention to the smell of your soap, shower gel, or shampoo. Listen to the water and other sounds. Feel the water running over your body, your hands shampooing your scalp, or the sensations of washing your body. See what you take in with your eyes. If some shampoo accidentally lands in your mouth, notice the taste. When thoughts try to distract you, like your to-do list or worrying about your infant as a teenager, take a deep breath and redirect your attention to the sensory experience of the shower: smell, touch, sound, sight, and taste. Do this for five or 10 minutes.

You can choose any activity you want to explore savoring. It may be a baby or non-baby related situation. If your baby creates pleasant sensations for you, practice paying attention to what it feels like when you look at them, touch them, or smell them, only after you've put them in clean clothes. Give them an arm or belly massage with soothing lotion and experience what you notice with your senses.

I like to practice with washing the dishes. When I attend to the full sensory experience of doing the dishes, it's pleasant. I notice the scent of the dish soap, the feel of the water rushing over my hands, and the sight of the bubbles as they appear and vanish. Zen meditation master Thich Nhat Hahn has said, "If you're not enjoying washing the dishes, then you're probably not paying attention to what you're doing."

To practice this exercise, pick an activity you experience multiple times a week like the ones mentioned above. Focus your attention on the sensory awareness of the activity. If your mind starts to wander to other thoughts or internal feelings whether positive or negative, bring your awareness back to the sensory experience of the moment you're in. Whatever happens, do not judge yourself or become self-critical. Just gently return your attention to your experience of your five senses: smell, touch, sound, sight, and taste. At the end of 5 or 10 minutes, release your attention from the activity you've chosen, take a few deep breaths, and resume your day.

✎ Note-icing Your Experience

While sitting quietly, you may want to explore the following questions. If you like to keep a journal, this would be a good time to write down your answers to reflect on later.

❋ What did you notice about your sensory experience of the activity you chose?

❋ What did you notice about how you felt before the exercise and how you feel now? Were there changes you were aware of at different points in the exercise?

❋ If thoughts and emotions distracted you, what was it like to attempt to redirect your attention to your senses? Were there differences in how easy or difficult it was to do this during this exercise?

❋ What did you learn from this exercise about savoring and how you can use it to stress less and live better?

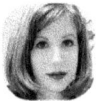

Megan's Mindful-ish Moment: FOMO and Parenting IRL

"That's so five minutes ago." This modern-day proverb, introduced in the original, feature-film version of *Buffy the Vampire Slayer*, was commonly used hyperbolically when I was growing up. It was funny because it was so true and untrue at the same time. Trends did come and go quickly, but not *that* quickly.

Today, the saying is no longer an exaggeration. Teens, tweens, and many adults feel chained to their electronic devices because five minutes is an eternity in the world of social media. Being five minutes behind renders one clueless, out of the loop, disregarded. The drive to stay current is so strong that my 13-year-old nephew refuses to go anywhere without wi-fi. Many people feel that social media can be a source of stress and anxiety, but the fear of missing out (FOMO) prevents them from cutting the digital apron strings.

FOMO, like so many trappings of our modern world, is the enemy of mindfulness. This may seem counterintuitive; after all, staying current on our devices 24/7 seems to be all about existing in the present moment. But anything that causes us to frenetically check up on a virtual existence that blocks out real experiences and sensations cannot be compatible with mindfulness. I'm not saying that social media, texting, and other forms of instantaneous information gathering are evil, per se. They can be a way to stay in touch, a source of inspiration, and an important marketing tool for businesses and individuals. Having sort-of-human contact and information immediately available and at our fingertips has unquestionably made life easier; however, FOMO, that ever-present fear of abandonment, has made it much more difficult as well.

FOMO as a catchphrase is relatively new. As a feeling, it is as old as time. I fell victim to it long before there was an acronym for it. The neighborhood where I lived for most of my childhood and adolescence was what you might call "suburban meets rural." On one side of a country road, there were a series of cul-de-sacs where people, including my family, lived on well-maintained three-to-nine acre plots of land. On the other side of the road was a field of cows. I was an only child, and most of my friends lived in town, much too far away for me to walk or ride my bike to their houses. I spent a lot of time on the phone and, after we got internet access, emailing and instant messaging, but physically, I was often isolated from other young people. I recall often looking out the window toward the empty horizon, imagining a city skyline and the glow of millions of lights. I had this fervent, uncontrollable feeling that everyone except me was at some fabulous party, having the time of their lives.

This, of course, was not the case. I did talk to a fair number of people my age, all of whom claimed to be as bored as I was. It was the 1990s, after all, so perpetual apathy was fashionable. Plus, my town was pretty boring. As recurrent as my party-exclusion fantasy was, FOMO still didn't affect me nearly as much as it does teenagers today. It did drive me to seek out any non-sports-related extracurricular activity I could find, and this overcommitment of myself sometimes did cause unnecessary anxiety.

FOMO started affecting me more during my twenties, in the age of social media proliferation. Then I discovered that girls' cattiness doesn't always disappear after high school; rather, mean girls grow up to become mean women. Even though we are well out of adolescence and supposed more emotionally mature, being excluded hurts. As inescapable as it can be, social media can intensify that pain. It must be so much worse for teenagers, for whom momentary trauma seems like it will last forever.

It may seem too early to talk about social media's role in our children's lives. Then again, I recently watched a Youtube tutorial in which a four-year-old teaches us how to use makeup to turn ourselves into unicorns. Thankfully, such digital precocity is still an exception rather than a rule, and even those of us engaged in early parenting have children who are still too young to feel the pull of the virtual world. But how long will that remain the case? Judging by how quickly the past five years have flown by for me, I'm guessing it won't be long. Before we know it, our children's peers will be conducting much of their social lives virtually, and schools will probably have an even greater online presence in the future than they do today. Does anyone want their child to be socially clueless and unable to do her homework? So, most of us will finally let our children have accounts on Twitter, Instagram, Snapchat, or whatever other social media interface has emerged in the next decade or so. (Facebook, apparently, is only for "old people.")

I quake with fear to contemplate that someday, my daughter could measure her worth by how many Instagram likes she receives. We can't let that happen to our kids, but what can we do to ensure that they don't become slaves to the digital world?

First of all, we can recognize that many young people have a love-hate relationship with social media. Many wish that they could reduce their social media usage or shut down their profiles entirely, but FOMO prevents them from doing so. Don't ever feel guilty for limiting your child's screen time, now or later. Whether they realize it or not, kids need boundaries and limits. Although, when they get older, they may complain and accuse you of "ruining their lives," don't succumb to their demands for greater access to their digital devices. If your child does miss out on "liking" his friend's Instagram post, he can always blame you and thus avoid accusations of being a bad follower.

Another way to keep your child free of social media's thrall is to make sure she has plenty of real-life social outlets. Trust me; there will be days when plunking your toddler down in front of some screen will seem much more appealing than carting her back and forth to Mommy and Me, Little Gym, Kindermusic, playgroups, and a plethora of other child-friendly activities. Your child may even seem to prefer the screen, too. I've seen a video of a three-year-old crying because her parents turned off the virtual animals on television so they could take her to see real animals at the zoo. At the moment, a toddler may care more about what happens on *Puppy Dog Pals* than an indeterminate and uncertain future anywhere else. I can't promise she will remember any particular outing for the rest of her life, but I can say with reasonable certainty that the zoo trip will have much more of an impact on her than an entire afternoon of Disney Junior programming. Similarly, your adolescent may drag his feet getting to extracurricular activities, but he is much likelier to remember making the game-winning goal in the soccer game than being the first person to know, via social media, that Tanner kissed Riley.

The final recommendation I have for you is to introduce mindfulness to your child at an early age, ideally before she becomes caught up in a barrage of social media. Children as young as four can learn mindfulness; you can refer to books like *The Mindful Child* for ways to practice mindfulness with your child. Luca enjoys "quiet sitting," especially because she gets to practice "noisy sitting" afterward!

Just like you, your child can also benefit from several ways to informally practice mindfulness. I don't know your child, so I can't tell you which of these ways will work best for him or her. That will be up to you. But I can tell you what informal mindful activities seem to be working well with Luca.

Luca is enrolled in Montessori school, which emphasizes what we used to call "kinesthetic learning," learning by doing. This fosters participation at the moment by manipulating materials rather than sitting still and listening to a lecture. Private schools, especially accredited Montessori programs that extend through the elementary grades like the one Luca attends, are often prohibitively expensive. Fortunately, you can find many resources that will help you integrate Montessori practices in your own home, if you so choose.

Anyone who knew me in high school will probably not believe I am going to say this, but I highly recommend getting your little one involved in sports. This can include any activity involving movement, from t-ball to cheerleading to horseback riding. Luca, for her part, currently takes gymnastics, dance, soccer, and swim lessons in the summer. I recommend that your child starts at an early age with minimal pressure, so he or she can experience the joy of movement without too much awareness of being more or less skillful than others. In addition to the benefits most of us have heard about, including teaching the value of teamwork, perseverance, and a healthy lifestyle, sports promote mindfulness in the form of greater mind-body awareness. They also teach us that we may not succeed in every endeavor, and how to overcome failure.

Finally, perhaps the best way to raise a mindful, in real life child is to practice and model mindfulness yourself. Children pick up on a lot more than we suspect. Even fetuses in the womb are affected by their mothers' stress. Luca, like many young children, can handle unrealistic, over-the-top conflict—like T-rexes eating people and witches placing death-curses on infant princesses—without batting an eye. She knows that's "just TV." But if one person she loves raises their voice in anger at another, she becomes concerned and unsettled. Conversely, modeling mindfulness and loving kindness will help your child feel protected and content.

Less is More

In my therapy sessions with clients, I openly talk to them about how less can be more. Initially, they are reluctant to consider this and want to continue multitasking and overdoing. They want to believe that the more they get done, the better and more successful they'll feel. Unfortunately, the opposite is often true. Women who do too much enter therapy because their lives feel out of control and they think they are failing because they aren't able to do anything the way they'd like to.

This is particularly true for many of the families I see with infants and young children. Although they know that caring for young children requires much effort and energy, they are frequently over-scheduled and overwhelmed. Rather than focusing their attention and effort on what matters to them and feeling good about it, they report feeling exhausted, short-fused, irritable, and unhappy. Their emotional pitcher is empty.

From a health psychology perspective, I explain to them that periods of energy expenditure must be followed by periods of restoration to function optimally. Also, symptoms of depression, anxiety, and other health conditions are more likely to occur when you have no reserve. Since most of my clients come to see me when they're in distress, they're willing to do whatever it takes for them to feel better. They take inventory of the things they're doing that they can let go of or let others care for temporarily. They learn to do less so they will have the energy they need for themselves, their babies, and their families. They stop being picky about how things get done and learn to be grateful for not having to do it all.

But when they start feeling better, many resume their overdoing and feel worse again. I've had dozens of new moms come in and tell me after a week or two of feeling better that they don't know what happened that caused them to feel worse again. Usually, they describe a day or two that they decided to spend most of the day doing errands from sunup to sundown. They may have stayed up too late for a few nights, getting things done around their house that they wanted to do, but didn't have to be done. They may have gone wild over their child's birthday party, or having guests stay the weekend, or telling their partner that they can spend the weekend doing what they want and they'll oversee what's happening at home.

By this time in our conversation, they realize that they've overdone it and done themselves in unintentionally. Suddenly, their awareness changes. They understand that they can choose to overdo it and keep feeling worse, or go back to doing less and continue to feel better. For most, this is an ongoing challenge, but as they experience the benefits of not overdoing, they decide it's worthwhile.

Sequential Living

Sequential living refers to a term I developed to describe living your life one phase at a time without trying to do too many things at once. Like savoring, it teaches us to focus on what we're doing with our attention and sensory awareness rather than multitasking and spreading ourselves thin. After giving birth to her second child and trying to expand her business simultaneously, one of my clients reported feeling stressed and burned out. Instead of being happy about either her child or business, she felt she was failing at both. Knowing this was her last child, she wanted to enjoy time with her baby and savor the moments with him. However, her guilt about not working more on her business made it impossible for her to enjoy either.

In counseling, we talked about her having an infant and 2-year-old, and how she might want her family to be her priority because her children were young and she did not want to miss out on their early years. She said that she enjoyed the time she spent at home being a mom to her two boys. As her guilt diminished, she realized how fortunate she was to be able to focus on her sons while keeping her business stable and growing. Later, when her boys were older, she could make different choices if she wanted, dedicating greater time and energy to expanding her business. Although this was a hard decision for her, she knew it was the right one.

The idea of "sequential living" freed her from the stress of worrying that she was constantly falling short of doing well at home or work. She let the employee who she'd put in charge during her maternity leave step in and do some of the things she'd normally have done. Her employee welcomed expanding her role. It was a win-win.

Recognizing that we don't have to do it all at once—that we can make sequential choices about our lives and what's most important along the way—allows us to savor the phase of life we're in and enjoy important moments that will not come again. Still, many of us experience "time starvation," meaning that we fear we don't have enough time to do the things we want. When we think this way, it leads to feeling overwhelmed and stressed. With sequential living, we trust that there will be enough time to do what we desire most if we don't squeeze too much into too short a time. Rather than feeling overwhelmed and frantic, we can put our attention towards what's most important at the time, allowing us to stress less and live better.

Mindful-Minis for Savor the Moment: If You're Pressed for Time

* Practice mindful eating. Take one bite of food at a time and chew it thoroughly before you take the next one.

* Take the dog outside or go for a walk for at least five minutes and notice how the air feels against your skin, what scents you notice, like flowers or burning leaves, and the sights and sounds you take in.

* Close your eyes and spend five minutes paying attention to the sensation of sound. If your awareness strays to sensations other than sound, bring it back to what you hear as you listen.

* Practice the sensation of touch when you're folding the laundry. Notice what different fabrics feel like by touching them with your hands or rubbing them against your cheek.

* When you're brushing your teeth in the morning and evening, notice different sensations of taste, touch, sound, smell, and sight.

* Look out your window or examine a piece of art in your home for five minutes to explore the sensory experience of sight.

Motherhood and Savoring the Moment

Early motherhood offers many opportunities to savor sensory awareness. Unfortunately, many of us get tuned in to negative sensory experience, like hearing our baby cry or fuss, and find it difficult to shift our attention to positive or neutral sensations. However, by the second month or so when our baby smiles at us, this occurs naturally without much effort. Think of how you feel after it's been cloudy for a couple of weeks, but suddenly, the sun comes out. Paying attention to positive sensations improves our mood and makes life more satisfying.

While pregnancy and postpartum are a time of great upheaval, there is much to be savored too. I thought of how food never tasted as good as during my second trimester and how my baby's skin felt soft as rose petals. Looking at my daughter's changing expressions or watching her explore whatever grabbed her attention could make me giggle. I savored the peaceful look on her face when she slept. Her cooing and laughing were delightful to hear. It was pleasant to smell the Dreft laundry soap I used to wash her clothes and the baby powder or lotion we put on her after her bath. Many experiences could be savored when I let go of my anxiety about what was next or how I'd get through it and instead, directed my sensory awareness to the moment I was in.

Why Practice Savoring?

When we savor the moment we're in, our perception of experience changes. In many of his books, Dr. Deepak Chopra says that we step into the world of timelessness and flow with the current of life. Instead of catastrophizing about what's ahead, or dwelling on past mistakes, we are present to what is occurring now and the depth and breadth it offers. It took me a long time to understand this concept, and it is one that I remind myself of repeatedly so I don't forget.

I remember when my daughters were teenagers and wanted to talk to me and if I didn't stop what I was doing, the moment passed and my chance to be emotionally present and connected with them slipped by. Whatever I'd convinced myself was more important than listening to them wasn't. I didn't fully understand that the only moment we have is the one we're in, and that once this moment is over, it will not come again.

So, what does this have to do with motherhood? Everything! By learning to savor the positive sensations we have and share with our infants, we are more likely to enjoy our time with them and they with us. Savoring facilitates bonding and closeness, giving us the energy and stamina to cope with the miraculous and life-altering changes of pregnancy, postpartum, and early motherhood. In the next chapter, we'll learn more about how to keep our minds present-focused and clear. Read on.

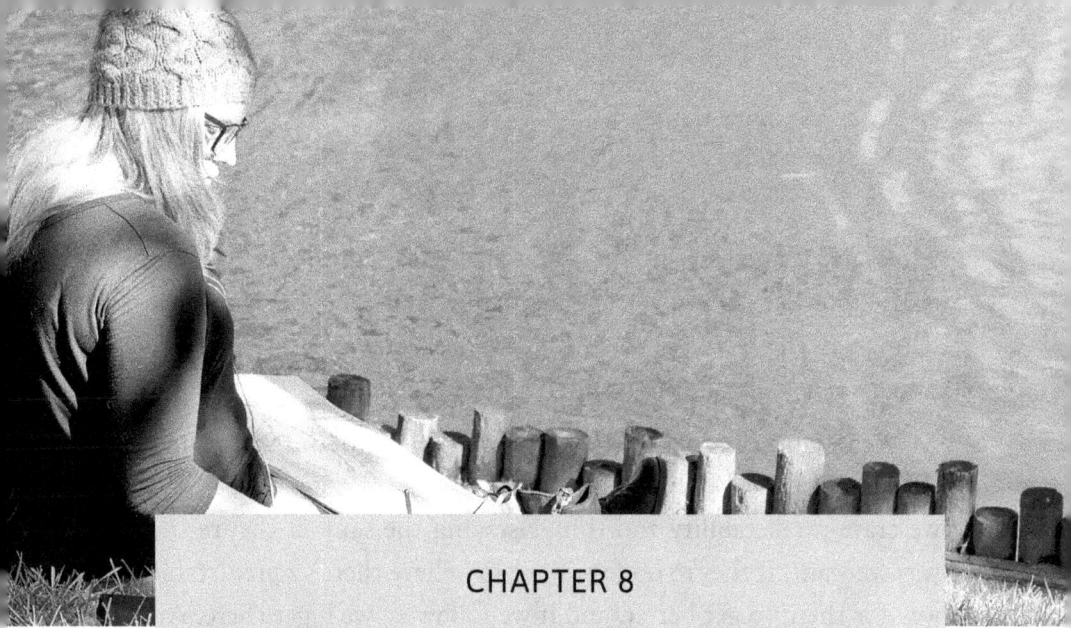

CHAPTER 8

SETTLE YOUR THOUGHTS
The Power of Letting Go

The first three skill sets in this book are about learning to stress less and live better by directing your attention to where you want it to go. The goal of this set of skills is to teach you how to notice your thoughts and let them pass without getting too attached to them. In class, we practice the exercises that involve focusing on our breath, bodies, or sensory experience first because before you can let go of unpleasant or disturbing thoughts, you must be able to direct your attention more skillfully than we are used to doing. If noticing what's happening in our bodies and sensory experience requires time and effort, learning to notice and then release our thoughts takes even more practice and persistence.

Others have compared the mind to a muscle and said that we need to strengthen it through regular mindfulness practice so that we don't get carried away and start imagining that because we have

139

a thought, it's necessarily true. Only the lived experience of an event or situation can inform you about whether your thoughts have been telling you the truth. In class, I talk about "letting life inform you" rather than believing that your thoughts are facts.

Remember, we spend 80% of our time living in the future, and 20% of our time dwelling on the past. I think this happens because we crave predictability and things staying the same if they're the way we want. If they're not, we want to believe there's a predictable way for them to get better, and if we follow it, we'll get there. An example of this is being a good person and working hard, expecting that this will bring us the things we deserve. However, life has many twists and turns, and if we get too attached to things working out a certain way, we may suffer and experience dis-ease.

Many of the thoughts we have about bad things happening are worse than what occurs. This is what brings many clients into psychotherapy. While their life circumstances may be stressful, they've become convinced that they will never get better or be able to enjoy life again. They dwell on how hopeless life has become, and how inadequate they feel. They ruminate continuously over their negative thoughts about the future or past, which intensifies their distress, anxiety, and depression.

As we start to explore how self-talk, or thoughts, may be interfering with their health and their ability to get better, I introduce the idea that thoughts are not facts, and that their thoughts only seem convincing because they keep repeating them. No one is likely to feel good if their head is filled with negative and self-defeating thoughts, which are common symptoms of anxiety and depression, as well as causes. First, they learn how to notice their thoughts. Next, they practice letting go of the ones that are not confirmed by experience. Since this can be a complicated idea, let's explore it through our skills practice.

📄 EXERCISE

Five-Minute Noting Our Thoughts Exercise

From my lived experience studying and teaching mindfulness, I believe that the ideas in this skill set are most easily understood through doing. So, let's practice the next exercise: Noting Our Thoughts.

This exercise can be practiced whenever you have a few free moments that are undisturbed and allow you to direct your attention to your thoughts. The goal of this exercise is not to notice the content of your thoughts, but to notice how they come and go. A related goal is not to get stuck on a single thought but to observe how they change. Doing this exercise often helps clarify this idea.

First, close your eyes and take three deep breaths. Notice where you experience the breath most strongly in your body at this moment. It may be around your lips and nostrils, or with the rise and fall of your chest, or the rise and fall of your belly. Do this for one minute.

Next, direct your attention to the thoughts that enter your mind. When you have a thought, you can say, "thought" to yourself, or imagine yourself making a checkmark in your mind, or count them as they occur. Do this for three minutes. Do not get hung up in the content or meaning of your thoughts. Note how they appear and then are gone.

Once you've noted your thoughts for a few minutes, release your attention from your thoughts, and redirect your attention back to your physical presence in the room. Notice feelings of your upper torso, lower torso, arms, legs, hands, feet, neck, shoulders, the front of your face, and the back of your head. You may want to wiggle or gently stretch, and if your eyes are closed, open them.

✐   *Note-icing Your Experience*

While sitting quietly, you may want to explore the following questions. If you like to keep a journal, this would be a good time to write down your answers to reflect on later.

* ❋ What did you notice about your experience of noting your thoughts? What was it like to not cling to them?

* ❋ What did you notice about how you felt before the exercise and how you feel now?

* ❋ What was it like to attempt to notice your thoughts without thinking about them? Did this get easier as the exercise progressed?

* ❋ How can you take what you learned in this exercise to help you stress less and live better?

Thoughts are NOT Facts

Many mindfulness teachers say that thoughts are NOT facts, but "mental events" that occur in our minds. At first, I was unable to understand what they were talking about. What is a mental event? How can they say thoughts are NOT facts? Certainly, my thoughts are true. While they may not be true for someone else, they're true for me, otherwise, why would I think them?

Through mindfulness practice, I gradually understood what they were saying. If I could learn to observe and direct my attention to my breath, my body, and my sensory experience, maybe I could learn to do the same with my thoughts. Once this occurred to me, I learned to pay attention to what I was thinking in a new way. For example, I might think that one of my friends was upset with me if I hadn't heard from them in a while, but instead of developing an elaborate story about what was happening, I simply noticed the thoughts I was having.

I observed that I would have many different thoughts about the same experience depending on how I felt at that moment. Although the situation was still the same, my thoughts about it weren't. With skill, it became easier to observe my thoughts as an object of attention rather than getting carried away with them. I learned that thoughts come and go and are not fixed and unchanging. An exercise we'll practice later in this chapter is called Observing Our Changing Thoughts; we learn to be aware of our thoughts and how they change.

Buddhist teachers say that our thoughts have a "sticky" quality, meaning we can easily become attached to them, and our attachment leads us to believe our thoughts accurately reflect reality. However, just because we think something doesn't make it true. Remember the story from earlier in this book about Buddha and how he realized that man created his suffering by the way he thought about things. Like Buddha, we can learn to stop this by observing or witnessing our thoughts instead.

Becoming the Witness

Another way in which mindfulness training teaches us to view our "thoughts as mental events," and not get carried away with them or become convinced that they are true, is the skill of "becoming the witness." When I first listened to Deepak Chopra explain this, I had no clue what he was talking about. After many years of study and practice, this skill has become invaluable to me, even if I don't always succeed.

Like noting our thoughts, "becoming the witness" requires us to step back from whatever we are experiencing in our thoughts, feelings, and bodily sensations, and observe what's happening like someone who is objectively witnessing what's occurring from outside of us. No, I'm not talking about anything weird. What I'm saying is that rather than getting caught up in your thoughts, feelings, and sensations, you learn to direct your attention to noticing your thoughts as an outside observer would. Imagine yourself as a TV broadcaster describing what's going on to your viewing audience, or a sports announcer relaying the plays in a game.

Here's an example from another teacher: Byron Katie. Katie describes an incident in which a mom is sitting outside on her porch waiting for her children to come home. It's early spring, the sun is shining, the flowers are growing, the birds are singing, and her body is experiencing many pleasant sensations UNTIL she starts thinking about her boys coming home. Then she has thoughts about how her older son will torment her younger son and that her younger son's self-esteem will be ruined. This leads her to think about how her younger son will never amount to anything, and her older son will become a bully. Now she is no longer enjoying pleasant sensations in her body, but feeling stressed and apprehensive. She is also sad and unhappy, imagining each of her sons' unfortunate futures.

In "becoming the witness," we learn to observe our thoughts, feelings, and sensations as they occur and describe the sequence of mental, emotional, and physical experiences we're having while trying not to get too caught up in them. Like Katie's description above, we note what's occurring in our minds and bodies without stirring up the "tigers within," or activating unpleasant thoughts, feelings, and sensations that threaten calm and wellbeing.

──────────────── 📄 EXERCISE ────────────────

Observing Our Changing Thoughts

Like the previous exercise, the intent of "Observing Our Changing Thoughts" is to notice thoughts and let them go without becoming attached. We learn to be the observer who can loosen their stickiness and stop treating them as facts. As in the above story of the mom sitting outside on a beautiful day while dreading her sons coming home and what she expects will happen, we witness the thoughts we're having and do not let them carry us away into some story that may or may not occur. We never know with 100% certainty what is going to happen in the future until it occurs.

Let's try another exercise to make this clearer. Start by finding a place where you can sit or lie comfortably, and not be interrupted for the next 10 minutes. Once you sit or lie down, take a few deep breaths in and out, and notice where you experience your breath most strongly in your body at this moment. It may be around your lips and nostrils, or the rise and fall of your chest, or the rise and fall of your belly. Whatever happens is fine. There is no right or wrong way to do this exercise.

Next, begin to picture your thoughts as clouds passing through the sky or leaves floating down a stream or waves peaking and diminishing on the ocean. Each time a thought comes to mind, picture it coming into view and then going away when another thought appears. Some of my students like to use the image of the sun rising and setting, or the changing weather. Whatever image works for you, use it because this is your experience. Once you've picked an image in your mind, direct your attention to noticing when you have a thought and then let it go. The intention of this exercise is to become aware that although thoughts change, the observing or witnessing part of you is always there and can be called upon to notice what's happening in your mind without getting hijacked by your thoughts.

After about 10 minutes, release the image you've been using and redirect your attention to your physical presence in the room. Notice feelings of your upper torso, lower torso, arms, legs, hands, feet, neck, shoulders, the front of your face, and the back of your head. You may want to wiggle or gently stretch and if your eyes are closed, open them.

✎ *Note-icing Your Experience*

While sitting quietly, you may want to explore the following questions. If you like to keep a journal, this would be a good time to write down your answers to review later.

❋ What was it like for you to observe your changing thoughts as clouds passing through the sky or whatever image you used? Were you able to become aware of your thoughts without getting carried away with them? Did you experience yourself as the observer or witness?

❋ What did you notice about how you felt before the exercise and how you feel now? Were there changes you noticed during the exercise?

❋ What was it like to attempt to notice your thoughts without thinking about them? Were there differences in how easy or difficult it was to do this from start to finish?

❋ How could you take what you have learned from this experience, and use it to stress less and live better?

Motherhood, Worry, and Fearful Thoughts

Whether you're pregnant or postpartum, most moms worry about their baby's health, whether their child is developing normally or not, imagined or actual harm coming to their child, their child's future, how they'll be as a mom, how they compare to other moms, and if they're a good enough mom. These worries are heightened by our access to social media and seeing pictures of other smiling moms with their smiling babies, when at the moment you feel overwhelmed, distressed, and that you're abnormal because you don't have this "Hallmark card" life. In reality, motherhood is hard work—a mix of joy and sorrow, loss and gain, happiness and despair. With time, most moms gain a sense of confidence and trust in themselves, regardless of the challenges they face. They will be able to meet them and successfully handle them.

Of course, this is a learning process that happens over time, and it is normal to feel worried and lack confidence when you start on the journey of pregnancy, postpartum, and early motherhood. However, getting carried away with catastrophizing about worries and fearful thoughts can interfere with positive mood and our ability to deal with life stressors. That's why pregnancy and postpartum are a good time to build your mindful stress-reduction muscle with skills like the ones in my program, Stress Less, Live Better. By practicing the exercises mentioned earlier in this chapter, you can have less worry, and manage fearful thoughts without them controlling you so you can enjoy early motherhood more.

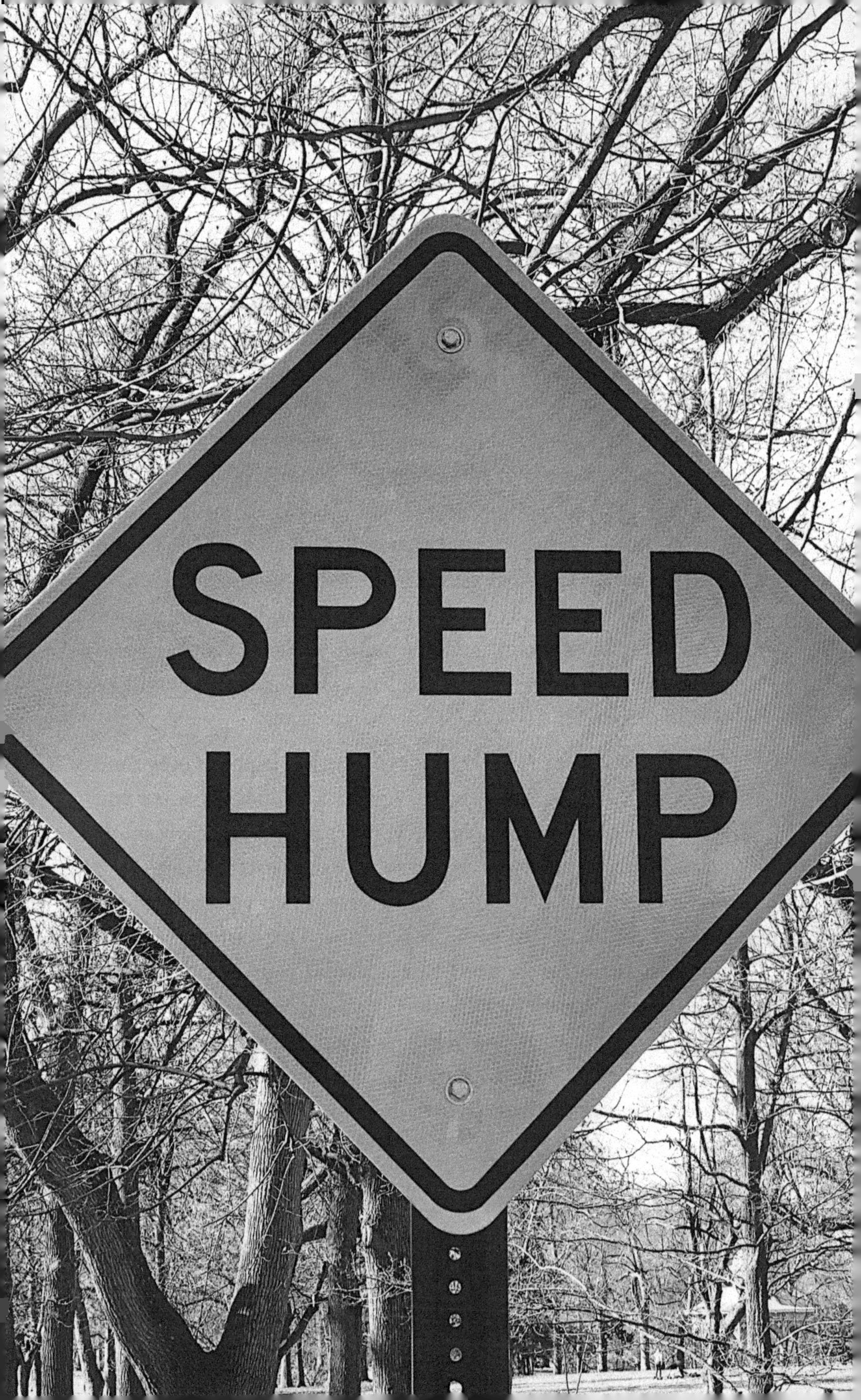
SPEED
HUMP

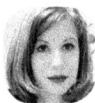

Megan's Mindful-ish Moment: Advice in the Internet Age

If you are a Millennial, or a tail-end member of Generation X, you were probably subjected to several school lessons concerning internet usage. I was in middle school when my school acquired internet access. The teachers warned us about all the misinformation available online and taught us how to distinguish between a reliable and unreliable source. What I gleaned from that lesson was this: a blog is an unreliable source. As I progressed in school and the internet advanced, I learned that certain material might be reliable for general knowledge but is inappropriate for citing in an academic paper. The major point of that lesson was this; scholarly journals are good sources, Wikipedia is not.

I assume we all know not to believe everything we read on the internet. WebMD has valid information but is not an acceptable substitute for a diagnosis from a professional. If your child has questions about sex, make sure she is asking you and not Yahoo Answers. This is all common sense by now. But as many of you know firsthand, common sense can tend to fly out the window when you become a new parent. I know parents raised children successfully for a couple of million years before the advent of the internet. But in many of my own internal battles between technology and so-called maternal instinct, technology usually wins.

During my baby's first year of life, I scoured the internet for answers to any question I had about her. Instant solutions were available with a few keystrokes, whereas 20 years earlier, I would have had to call a friend with kids, my mother, or a doctor, or even go to an actual library and check out a book. And you know us introverts. We aren't always in the mood for having a telephone conversation or leaving the house. Before we became parents, my

husband and I had consulted blogs and message boards for answers
to important questions, such as, "How do I keep my cat from peeing
on the floor?" (We tried everything and none of the recommendations
worked, but we remained undeterred, figuring we just hadn't found
the right technique yet.)

When I became a parent, I turned to the internet again to
answer questions like, "Why won't my baby feed herself?" "How
much screen time is too much for an 8-month-old?" "What the
heck is this rash?" Eventually, I started to suspect that this method
of research was not going to be good enough. As much as we love
our fur babies, we love our human babies even more, so why would
we go through the same channels to get advice about children as
we do to get advice about pets? This is not a rhetorical question.
We do this because the internet has become the Supreme Source
of All Knowledge, and it is practically automatic to consult it. And
most of the time, why wouldn't you? Many people my age, myself
included, get almost all their news and current events information
online. Even Wikipedia, once the bane of professors everywhere,
is much more reliable and better-policed than it once was.

Because the internet, as a whole, seems so endless and omniscient,
it is easy to forget that it is also still a forum for absolutely anyone
to spout opinions that have no basis in reality. While the internet
has come a long way in many areas, some of the parenting sites are
still the cyber equivalent of the Wild West. The post you're reading
could be written by a middle-aged MD who has raised several
children, or it could be from an 18-year-old with the Grammarly
app, who has just come from posting an alternative definition of
"thot" on urban dictionary. For that matter, it could have been
written by an internet troll whose only experience with parenting
consists of living in his mother's basement. Having temporarily
forgotten what I learned at 13, I found myself at 33, trying to

Ferberize my infant, and sobbing because some woman on a message board said that parents who let their babies cry alone for 10 minutes are cruel, inhumane, and should be reported to Child Services. Feeling more rational, but a bit uncharitable in the light of the following day, I thought, "This woman will still be co-sleeping with her 15-year-old while her undersexed partner sleeps in the guest room." Now I am more mindful and try not to answer judgment with judgment. Sleeping arrangements are a personal choice, and I respect whatever choice parents make for themselves and their children. (Just between us, though, I still suspect that Brangelina's split may have had at least a little to do with their habitual practice of co-sleeping with all six children at once.)

Whether our questions concern development, behavior, or health, I think every parent wants to know, "Is my child normal?" If you ask everyone, which is essentially what you're doing when you go online, someone out there is going to say no. If I go out on a busy sidewalk and ask everyone who passes if I look like a monkey, someone is going to say yes. That doesn't make it true (I hope). This example might seem silly, but it illustrates an important point. Do not seek out answers to serious questions about your child from random people online. You know your child better than they do. If you are concerned, schedule an appointment with an expert, like a doctor or psychologist. In the meantime, try to refrain from reading what people say about your child's condition on message boards or comments sections below articles. If you must go online, please consult specific, trusted sources rather than doing indiscriminate Google searches like I once did.

Don't get me wrong, I still receive plenty of parenting advice— some unsolicited, some sought-after. To me, it would have been impossible to survive potty-training a few years ago without three books and countless expert and non-expert opinions. After all, polite society will probably forgive you your incontinent cat with a "behavioral, not medical" problem. They might not feel that way about an elementary schooler with the same behavior. I probably absorbed more information than I needed about potty-training. For instance, I learned that some American children now arrive at kindergarten still wearing diapers, while in many other countries, children are toilet-trained as soon as they learn to walk. As with most subjects, there is no shortage of people who claim to know the best and only way to potty train. My husband and I considered the varied and often conflicting advice and tailored an approach that worked for our daughter and us.

Before I started practicing mindfulness, toilet-training would have been much more stressful. The sheer quantity and scope of the advice would have frazzled me. I would have had trouble adhering to one technique for a sufficient length of time. If one approach didn't work right away, I would have switched to another. This would have probably made for a confusing and upsetting transition for my daughter. Fortunately, I did practice mindfulness by then. I was able to stay in the moment, which made me more patient and able to deal with one challenge at a time.

Now I am better able to deal with both advice and judgment. I am a grown woman, and so are you, and we aren't obligated to take all the advice we are given! I will consider any recommendation and determine how and whether it will work for me in my situation. If I disagree with the advice, or don't think it will work for me, I let it go. I do my best not to dwell on it, second-guess my decision, or let it cause me undue anxiety. If someone wholly unconnected with me thinks some of my parenting practices will scar my child for life, I will take it with a grain of salt. I will wish that person well with their parenting journey but will agree to disagree.

I am far from worry-free, and am a constant work in progress as a parent. Perhaps you are, too. If you find yourself dealing with information overload, either internet-induced or otherwise, try Diane's exercise, "Observing Our Changing Thoughts," beginning on page 144.

How Normal Mom Worries Differ from Clinical Anxiety and OCD

These guidelines are based on my 30 years of clinical experience with psychological counseling and assessments of perinatal women with symptoms of anxiety and OCD. Remember, this book is not intended to offer clinical advice, and you should always consult a healthcare provider if you are concerned about having these symptoms. Asking a family member or friend with whom you have a confiding relationship to give you honest feedback about your concerns may be helpful too. For more clinical information, consult Postpartum Support International at www.postpartum.net or Karen Kleiman's Postpartum Stress Center at www.postpartumstress.com.

Besides the "baby blues" triggering at delivery, postpartum anxiety and OCD can also start then. The difference is that over time, usually 3 to 6 weeks, the "baby blues" go away while clinical anxiety and depression continue to get worse. By a mom's second or third month postpartum, and often when she returns to work, she will begin thinking that something isn't right. With so many changes occurring at once, women often put off seeking treatment or accepting that something could be wrong with their emotional health. Some women wait beyond the first year of their child's life when postpartum officially ends to get help. If their clinical conditions go un-or-undertreated, they usually get worse until they can't ignore them or they stumble along as best they can. For full recovery from clinical anxiety and OCD, treatment is required.

Here are some of the symptoms that, if they become worse with each passing week, you want to consult a healthcare provider for treatment. With clinical anxiety, you are likely to experience panic attacks, where your heart races, you feel out of control, or that you are having a heart attack, your breathing becomes shallow, you feel like you're going to pass out or start hyperventilating, and, in general, experience numerous unpleasant bodily sensations. Your stress reaction constantly triggers, and you are in a perpetual state of fight or flight. Because you are stressed out all the time, you are likely to have problems eating, sleeping, paying attention, concentrating, and feeling content. It's as if you sense danger lurking around every corner and feel like you can never let your guard down, and are convinced that if you stop being hyperalert, something bad will happen.

With clinical OCD, you have recurring anxiety-producing thoughts that won't stop. There may be worries about your baby's, your family's, or your health, and some catastrophe occurring. I've had moms who are convinced that their children have CP or some incurable, awful childhood illness. Other moms think they have cancer or another life-threatening disease. However, the most disturbing and distressful OCD thoughts are those in which moms have thoughts of harming their children. Unlike moms with postpartum psychosis, moms with clinical OCD are not at risk of harming their children because they know these thoughts are wrong and are repulsed by them. They are guilt-ridden and think they are the worst of all moms.

With effective treatment, postpartum anxiety and OCD are 99.9% curable. So don't wait. Talk to a health provider now. The sooner you get treatment, the sooner you'll feel better and enjoy your life again.

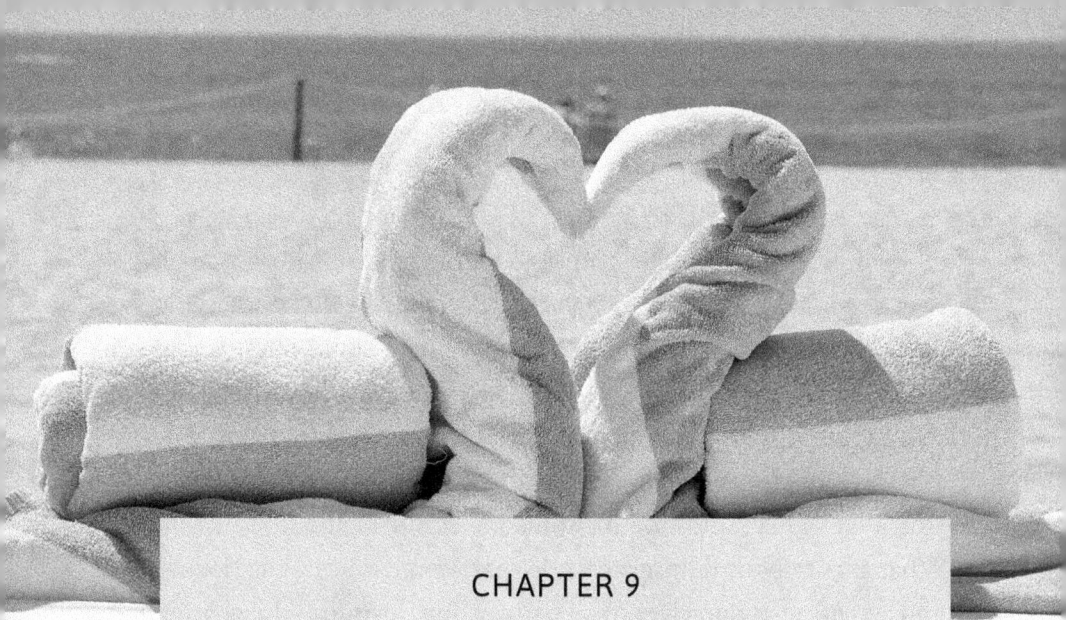

CHAPTER 9

SELF-COMPASSION ALWAYS

The Power of Acceptance

The final skill in my class is Self-Compassion Always. I put it last because I thought mindfulness was what students needed to learn most. Instead, I discovered that most women are painfully self-critical, evaluative, and rejecting of themselves. While they are willing to forgive others for their mistakes, and be gentle and patient with them, they are not to themselves.

Why is this when the women's movement is decades old? I think there are a couple of reasons. First, research on the female brain has shown that from the time their moms become pregnant with them, female hormones bathe their brains in chemicals that make them more focused on relationships. Likewise, their moms and other women have taught then, directly and indirectly, to be nice and put other people's needs above their own. Other love becomes a higher priority than self-love to girls and young women who are challenging the boundaries of traditional women's roles.

Self-acceptance or self-compassion is often lacking until women reach a point in their lives when they decide they are as deserving of their love and attention as the rest of their loved ones. Rabbi Hillel, in *Teachings of Our Fathers,* said, "If I am not for myself, who will be for me? If I am only for myself, what am I? If not now, when?" Singer, songwriter, and activist Melissa Etheridge put it this way: "There's no love for someone else if I can't love myself." What they're both talking about is that we must be caring, loving, and accepting of ourselves to be truly caring, loving, and accepting of others. How can we teach our loved ones to do this when we're rejecting and critical of ourselves?

There is great power in cultivating self-compassion and acceptance. Learning to accept yourself fully, with your strengths and flaws, can be reassuring and liberating. Once you learn to recognize your judging and evaluative self, and turn the volume down or talk back to self-critical remarks, you open yourself to more fully creating a life you desire. You start to feel supported and have more energy for yourself and others.

Self-acceptance doesn't mean that you stop doing your best. It means that as human beings, we make mistakes, and this is how we grow. It is allowing the lighter and darker parts of our nature to co-exist. It is treating yourself with respect and love always. Buddha said, "You, as much as anyone else, are deserving of your love." These next exercises will help you understand this skill better. Practicing them in your life will help them stick.

Noticing Your Negative Self-Talk

At first, students and counseling clients are unaware of the frequency and severity of their negative self-talk when they are feeling stressed, anxious, or depressed. All they realize is that they feel bad. As we begin to explore what they've been telling themselves by keeping a stress diary or observing their negative self-talk, themes begin to emerge, including:

* ❋ I'm not a good enough mom, daughter, or friend.

* ❋ Every time my life starts getting better, something bad happens.

* ❋ If you stop worrying about the future, bad things will happen.

* ❋ Because I'm not smart enough

* ❋ (you fill in the blank), I don't deserve a good life.

The list is endless.

--------------------- 📄 E X E R C I S E ---------------------

Noticing Your Negative Self-Talk Exercise

To help you tune into these messages, here's an exercise on observing negative thoughts and feelings you may have about yourself and your life. First, find a comfortable place in your home or office where you can reflect on the following questions for the next 10 minutes without being disturbed. You may want to take your journal with you to make some notes later. Next, gently and lovingly close your eye if you want, and begin to focus on your breath as it flows in and out of your body. Notice where you experience the breath most strongly in your body. It may be around your lips and nostrils, or in the rise and fall of your chest, or the rise and fall of your belly. Spend a moment or two following it from inhalation to exhalation. If thoughts, feelings, or bodily sensations distract you, return your attention to the breath.

Next, imagine a situation where you were stressed, anxious, or depressed, and notice the thoughts leading up to it or following this experience. For example, I was taking a mindfulness class recently with a new teacher and started feeling agitated and self-critical during an exercise on courage. It wasn't the exercise itself, but my thoughts comparing myself to the new teacher. I found myself thinking that she was doing better than I would have. When we finished, I realized that this was my negative voice shouting in my ear and set it aside, so it didn't torment me.

Keep mental notes of the negative remarks your "negative voice" said to you during the stressful, anxious, or depressive-producing situation in all the detail you remember. Once you've done this for a few minutes, redirect your attention to imagining yourself as a baby. Maybe you remember a family picture or video you've seen. Then picture you as an adult smiling at this sweet infant who's innocent and full of awe. A baby who deserves your love and all the best life can bring. Look at the baby and say, "I love you," picturing this in your mind for a few moments.

Finally, release your attention from you as an adult looking at your infant self and return your attention to your physical presence. Notice physical sensations of your upper torso, lower torso, arms, legs, hands, feet, neck, shoulder, the front of your face, and the back of your head.

You may want to wiggle or gently stretch, and if your eyes are closed, gently and lovingly open them.

✎ Note-icing Your Experience

While sitting quietly, you may want to explore the following questions. If you like to keep a journal, this would be a good time to write down your answers to think about later.

❋ What thoughts, feelings, and bodily sensations did you experience during this exercise?

❋ What did you notice about how you felt before the exercise and how you feel now? What did you notice when changes occurred?

❋ What was it like to picture yourself as a baby?

❋ What did you learn from this exercise about self-compassion?

Befriending Yourself

When we discuss self-compassion in class, I use a cartoon that pictures our negative and self-critical thoughts as the Judge, Jury, and Executioner inside our heads. What does this mean? I use these images to point out the harsh and derogatory comments women frequently make about themselves. First, we judge ourselves to be wrong or unworthy. Then we sentence ourselves to feeling bad and shamed. Finally, we punish ourselves with negative self-talk that erodes our self-esteem, health, and happiness.

What can we do about this? In individual counseling and classes, I talk about how women and others need to learn to befriend themselves. Most of us would never say the things to our friends or loved ones that we say to ourselves. Who would tell a loved one how badly he/she should feel for making a mistake or saying the wrong thing? Who would say to a friend, "You really suck," or "What's wrong with you anyway?"

Instead, we encourage our friends and loved ones with our support. Our opinion doesn't suddenly go from thinking they're wonderful to thinking they're awful like it can when we think about ourselves. We don't stop loving and start rejecting them. This is something we reserve for ourselves. What we need to do is treat ourselves with compassion and forgiveness like we would a friend, accepting that we are not perfect and that's okay. Yes, we may be able to do better next time, but making mistakes is human.

Another way to put this is that while our mistakes or poor choices may affect and influence us, we do not let them define who we are. When we choose to learn from our mistakes, we befriend ourselves by making

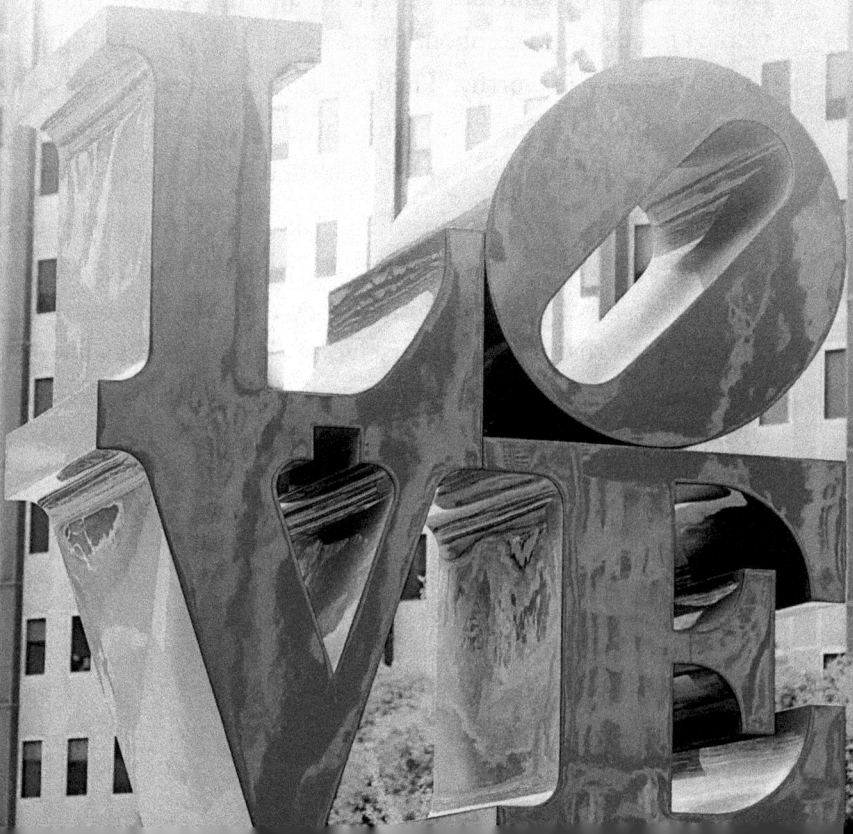

this choice rather than continuing to beat ourselves up with judging and negative self-talk. We learn to encourage ourselves and free ourselves from the repetitive cycle of being our own worst enemy.

In *The Lion King*, when Rafiki the mandrill speaks to Simba about seeing what happened as an experience he can learn from, and how the pride is suffering under his uncle's rule, Simba agrees to return. He overthrows his uncle and becomes the rightful king. Only once Simba overcame his guilt and feelings of unworthiness could he reach his full potential. In one of the final scenes, we see his father's spirit looking down on him and smiling with love and respect for the leader his son has become.

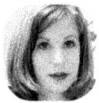

Megan's Mindful-ish Moment

Comparisons and Self-Compassion

This section is not directly related to pregnancy or parenting. It is, however, related to women in general, regardless of which life-stage we occupy. In my opinion, the drive to measure our successes against those of others can affect multiple facets of our lives, which is especially evident in the phenomenon of "competitive parenting." Furthermore, the lesson to be the best version of *yourself* (not better or worse than someone else) is something we will want to teach our children too. You're never too young to learn self-compassion.

One way we can start practicing self-compassion is by resisting the urge to compare ourselves with others, but this is easier said than done. My husband loves to say that I invariably adore television shows whose target demographic is 13-year-old girls. (He should not be one to talk, as he has the viewing taste of a 7-year-old with ADHD. I suspect he got Luca hooked on *The Amazing World of Gumball* for his selfish reasons. She is too young to be watching it, but I have felt at a disadvantage to criticize Dave for what *he* allows her to watch ever since she started singing the opening credits to *Orange is the New Black*, one of *my* favorite shows.)

Dave is partially correct. I confess to crying a little on the inside when the CW canceled *America's Next Top Model*, and the reboot is just not the same. Back in the days of scripted television, it was probably easier to recognize the divide between ourselves and the actors we watched. After all, for many of them, it was part of their job to look attractive. They also had makeup artists, fitness trainers, personal chefs, and a plethora of other image-makers to help them. I think most viewers knew this. We had shows like *Lifestyles of the Rich and Famous* and *Cribs* to show us that, despite what a certain magazine might have us believe, celebrities are not just like us.

Since the advent of reality television, I believe that it has become increasingly difficult to resist comparing ourselves to what we see. During the early days of reality TV, this might not have been so harmful. Looking back at the first few seasons of *The Real World*, it's astonishing just how average-looking those people were. But there has been a shift, so gradual and insidious that we might not have noticed. Now we are comparing ourselves to so-called "real" women with blindingly-white veneered smiles, fake hair, and eyelash extensions, who have been shellacked and spray-tanned and, possibly, starved within an inch of their lives to appear on *The Bachelor*.

Theoretically, I know that reality TV is about as real as Cheez Whiz and unicorns. In practice, I'm thinking, "Well, *some* of this must be real. I'm just not sure what and how much." And the reality franchises are not exactly forthcoming. In practice, I might binge-watch an entire season of *Top Model* and find myself thinking, "I don't look like that," which turns into "I should look like that," and then "JUST TELL ME WHAT I NEED TO DO TO LOOK LIKE THAT AND I'LL DO IT!" But then I turn off the devil-box and try to put these things in perspective.

I am not an 18-year-old model, nor do I aspire to be. I am married, and if I were not, I certainly think making myself physically beyond reproach to vie for a man along with a couple of dozen other women would probably not be the most practical way of "finding love." Most of us must procure and prepare our food, make a living using our wits rather than our looks, take care of families, and do any number of other things that are arguably better uses of our time than appearing on reality television. If we don't want to emulate these women in regards to the way they spend their time, why should we be expected to emulate the way they look?

If we are endeavoring to be more mindful, we need to stop comparing ourselves to other women, period, not just TV personalities, fashion magazine models, or Instagram influencers. Remember, mindfulness is about being aware of the present moment without judgment, and what is comparison if not another way of judging ourselves, usually unfavorably? Furthermore, mentally pitting ourselves against other women does not promote the sense of sisterhood that is so desperately needed in our current political climate. Being preoccupied with the way we look does not make us better wives, mothers, or friends. I recently read the following quote in a blog post by Liz Henry, and although it is about the no-makeup movement, it can apply more generally as well. She writes:

> If I meet up with a makeup-less friend, my first thought isn't, "Looks like your contour was set to

frump today." Nope, my first thought is, "Yay! I have
a friend!"

Look at yourself the way you would look at a friend, with compassion.
Now that I'm well out of high school, "hotness" does not even rate
on my list of desirable qualities in a friend. I would much prefer
she be kind, trustworthy, and a good listener. Your friends and
family probably feel the same way about you.

I'm not recommending that anyone (or, God forbid, myself)
refrain from the occasional media binge-fest. Nor am I suggesting
that we all constantly question and critique everything we see, as
it is annoying enough when *someone else* tries to deny you your
escapism (try watching *Gladiator* with someone with a doctoral
degree in Ancient European History). But I am challenging myself
to, afterward, be mindful of what messages I choose to take away
from what I watched.

Even if we manage to negotiate the gauntlet of beauty and
body comparisons, other dangers still lie ahead. As moms and
moms-to-be, we should be aware of the phenomenon of "mommy
comparisons." Logging onto Facebook can bum me out. It seems
as though everyone I ever knew has a picture-perfect family, a
fantastic, rewarding job, and has recently traveled to an exotic
location, either to relax in lavish style or to build schools and
dig wells.

Remember that people on social media platforms, like
Facebook, usually only show their best possible self. You probably
do it, too. Most of our acquaintances are not going to post
pictures of themselves immediately after waking up in the
morning, or wolfing down the mediocre takeout they ordered
last night. The average Facebook user is not going to write a
status update about the argument they just had with their partner,

their dissatisfaction with their job, or their fears and misgivings.

Sometimes I think people must be judging and thinking negative thoughts about me: that I am a bad parent or didn't live up to my potential. Right now, I'm thinking that you, dear reader, are saying, "Damn, that woman watches too much TV." In actuality, these are all my thoughts that I have internalized to the point that I believe that everyone else is thinking the same thing.

We may think someone has everything figured out, but do we ever consider that person may be thinking the same thing about us? April, the director of Luca's Montessori school, is about the same age as Dave and I, and has two children: one younger than Luca and one older. I know that she has practiced the Montessori philosophy with them since birth, and they always seem so friendly, polite, and well-adjusted. She also seems to possess an abundance of optimism and patience. She came up to Dave and me at the end of our most recent Parent Education night and said she appreciated us being there, and for being such supportive and involved parents. Dave and I feel that, to paraphrase Chris Rock, supporting your kid is a "s'posed-to-do" that we need not to be congratulated upon. Nevertheless, I appreciated April's sentiment. I said something to the effect of, "Are you kidding? You're the amazing parent here," and cited the reasons listed above. She said, "Are *you* kidding? I want to be you guys when I grow up!" Then we laughed because we are all supposedly grown-ups.

Be kind to yourself. In the unlikely event that someone is judging you harshly, remember that this is their problem, not yours. When you find yourself being your own worst critic, try the Loving Kindness Meditation that follows.

📄 EXERCISE

Loving-Kindness Meditation

Loving-kindness, or Metta meditation, is a practice designed to cultivate self-compassion. You'll want 10 to 15 minutes to practice in a quiet, comfortable place at home. This exercise is probably best done sitting to stay alert and awake. It is calming, but also energizing in a classroom or yoga studio when done with other students.

To begin, gently close your eyes, or leave them open if you like. Take in a few deep breaths and notice where your breath occurs most strongly in your body at this moment. It may be around your lips and nostrils, or in the rise and fall of your belly, or the rise and fall of your chest. See if you can follow it from inhalation to exhalation and back again. If thoughts, feelings, and sensations distract you, gently redirect your attention to your breath.

Then repeat the following words silently to yourself.

May I be at peace.

May my heart remain open.

May I know the beauty of my own true nature.

May I be healed.

May I be a source of healing to others.

Take a few deep breaths and let the words sink in before moving on.

Next, repeat the same words silently to yourself, but this time, make your loved ones the focus by saying these words.

May you be at peace.

May your heart remain open.

May you know the beauty of your own true nature.

May you be healed.

May you be a source of healing to others.

Take a few deep breaths allowing the words to sink in before moving on.

Next, choose someone you're having difficulty with, and extend loving kindness to them.

May you be at peace.

May your heart remain open.

May you know the beauty of your own true nature.

May you be healed.

May you be a source of healing to others.

Take a few deep breaths and let the words sink in before moving on.

Next, offer this meditation of loving kindness to all the people in your community by saying:

May we be at peace.

May our hearts remain open.

May we know the beauty of our own true nature.

May we be healed.

May we be a source of healing to others.

Take a few deep breaths and allow these words to sink in before moving on.

Finally, extend loving kindness to all living beings in our world, and this beautiful planet we call home with these words.

May all of us be at peace.

May all our hearts remain open.

May all of us know the beauty of our own true nature.

May all of us be healed.

May all of us be a source of healing to others.

Take a few moments to allow these words to sink in, and then return your attention to your physical presence in the room. Notice physical sensations of your body against the chair, sofa, or mat on which you're sitting. Notice sensations of your upper torso, lower torso, arms, legs, hands, feet, neck, shoulders, the front of your face, and the back of your head. You may want to wiggle or gently stretch, and when you feel ready if your eyes are closed, allow them to open.

Don't Take Things Personally

A related issue that can either diminish or strengthen our self-compassion is how we interpret what happens between us and others. Learning not to take things personally is one of Don Miguel Ruiz's Four Agreements. In his book, *The Four Agreements,* Ruiz gives principles to live by: "Always be impeccable with your word; Don't take things personally; Don't make assumptions; and Always do your best." Although each of these relates to self-compassion, clients and students report that learning not to take things personally, and become independent of the good opinion of others, has helped them most with self-compassion.

Here are some examples of taking things personally. You are spending time with a good friend who seems upset and annoyed.

You ask them what's bothering them and they get more ticked off. You assume it's something you said or did, and start to feel uneasy. The next day, your friend tells you she fought with her partner yesterday before you met, and wasn't ready to talk about it. It had nothing to do with you.

Another example students and counseling clients frequently report is being at a party and having the sense that someone took what they said the wrong way because the other person is short or seems annoyed. Instead of considering what may be going on for them, you assume you said or did something to them only to find out a few days later that their mom just got diagnosed with cancer. It had nothing to do with you.

In a backward way, taking things personally gives us a sense of greater control over our lives by thinking if we're responsible for someone feeling bad, we can fix it. However, how other people feel and act has much more to do with what's happening in their lives than us. When we stop worrying about what they think of us, we can see this more clearly. For most women, this is hard to do because of our need for approval and being liked. Many of us were raised to put others first and be people pleasers. The problem with this is that it frequently backfires on us.

Although it sounds counter-intuitive, by not taking things personally, we gain more control over ourselves and our relationships. How does this work? When we become able to say to ourselves that the way someone reacts has more to do with them than us, we begin to relax. We can listen more clearly to what the other person is saying without defending ourselves or worrying about what we're going to say next. We can be more likely to give them what they need without getting hung up on how we are.

📄 EXERCISE

Put More Joy in Your Life Exercise

When I see the word "joy," I sometimes feel pressured to come up with something that will make me ecstatically happy. This is not what I mean for you to do in this next exercise. Instead, the goal is to notice the small things in your life that make you feel good, like sitting in front of a picture window on a sunny day, and experiencing the warmth on your shoulders and neck (which is what I've been doing today). It's discovering what helps you feel warm and cozy, which is different for each of us. I recently had the experience of lamenting to someone my disappointment over another gray day, and she said, "I love gray days, crawling under my blanket, and enjoying a warm cup of tea." Don't make assumptions.

Finding little things in life that make you feel good is an important part of self-compassion, self-care, and mindfulness. When we engage in activities that make us feel good, we are self-compassionate by treating ourselves with appreciation. Our actions help refill our emotional pitcher so that we have the energy and strength we need to weather life's ups and downs. Likewise, they help bring our attention to the moment we're in, and how we can feel better, whether our current life is bumpy or smooth.

Here's the exercise. During the next week, experiment with what makes you feel good that doesn't involve anyone else. Make a list of five experiences that bring you joy and pleasant feelings. It might be spending 10 minutes of solitude drinking your morning coffee or tea. Perhaps you take 15 minutes before you pick up your kids from school to walk or be outside. Maybe you decide to phone a friend or listen to your playlist. At the end of the week, write down what you did and how you experienced it: feelings, thoughts, and bodily sensations. Then, review your responses. You can also track this on your phone or calendar.

If you've gotten out of the habit of doing things for yourself, or noticing what feels good to you, try these modifications. First, recall things you used to enjoy as a child or younger adult. I remember it felt great to lie on a beach towel in the sun. The warmth of the sun with the coolness of the spring breeze was delightful. Now, I like to sit on my deck with the sun on my face and a cool beverage in my hands, enjoying these sensations like when I was young. Give yourself 5 to 10 minutes to recall what used to bring you pleasant feelings. Try practicing some of these things in the next week. At the end of the week, make some notes about what you did and how you felt on paper or your phone. See what you notice.

The third option for this exercise is to note simple experiences that make you feel good for a week. Maybe you notice you spend 10 extra minutes making yourself lunch rather than grabbing it on the run. Perhaps you spend 15 minutes on a nice day to sit at the picnic table outside your office building to have lunch or take a break from your work. Notice how it feels when you're not rushing around or hurrying to get from one place to another. Maybe you get a call from a neighbor that she'll pick your child up from school and bring him back to her house for a playdate. Notice what that's like and how you feel. Notice the situations that create pleasant thoughts, feelings, and bodily sensations, and those that don't. Use these experiences to make a list of the little things that bring you joy for future use.

Gratitude

Gratitude is another piece of developing self-compassion. It includes feeling grateful for yourself and the wonderfulness of you. Helen Keller said, "What I am looking for is inside me. Not out there." Gratitude is an appreciation for your existence and how you have contributed to life. It is loving yourself fully and acknowledging both success and failure help us grow, shaping the person we become.

Here's a poem describing this by the 14th century Persian poet, Rumi.

THE GUEST HOUSE

This being human is a guest house. Every morning a new arrival.

A joy, a depression, a meanness. Some momentary awareness comes. As an unexpected visitor.

Welcome and entertain them all. Even if they're a crowd of sorrows who violently sweeps your house. Empty of its furniture.

Still, treat each guest honorably. He may be clearing you out. For some new delight.

The dark thought, the shame, the malice. Meet them at the door laughing. And invite them in.

Be grateful for whoever comes because each has been sent. As a guide from beyond.

Motherhood and Acceptance

Other than adolescence, early motherhood may be the second biggest challenge women face in continuing to feel good about themselves. While I thought that the generation of moms following mine would be less self-critical and more accepting of themselves, this has not occurred. Instead, moms today feel more pressured to be "perfect," and our digital age of comparing ourselves to everyone else has made things worse.

Another obstacle is that many women today work to support their families financially and so whether they are at work or home, they feel inadequate, and their self-esteem suffers. Because they can't commit 100% of their effort or energy as they did to their work pre-children, they feel they're failing at their jobs. Lacking the emotional stamina to be "super-mom" after a long day at work, they fault themselves for not being able to care for their children and homes in the ways they desire.

Stay-at-home moms have an equally rough time, but for different reasons. Since motherhood is still the most underpaid and devalued profession in the world, they often view themselves as not "contributing" to their families. Several clients have told me that it's uncomfortable for them to go to a work-related function for their partner or socialize with women who work outside their homes. When people ask them "What do you do," they say with shame, not pride, "I'm a stay-at-home mom."

Finally, women are more self-critical and judgmental of each other than men are, and this has gotten worse in the digital era. Driven by our insecurities and fears, we act like there's a single right way to give birth, feed our babies, etc. and that if we're not abiding by the status quo, then we're flawed. The way we talk about other moms and the rude remarks over the internet are NOT the way to treat each other.

As women, we must learn to be accepting of ourselves and each other to set an example for our children and everyone whose lives we touch. It is up to us to redefine motherhood so that it is more valued and respected. This change starts inside ourselves. Once we become self-compassionate and accepting of ourselves, we can extend this to others. Only then can we redefine motherhood in a kinder and gentler way.

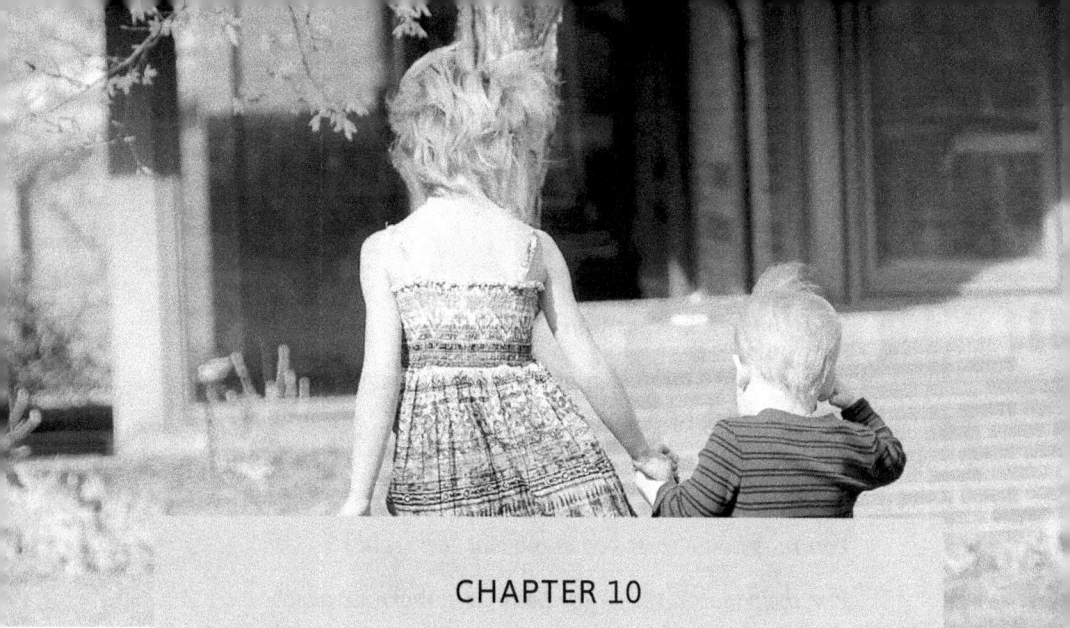

CHAPTER 10

CONCLUSION

Parenting and Accepting Our Children for Who They Are

In addition to accepting ourselves fully, learning to accept our children for who they are can be equally challenging. Before we have children, many of us imagine what we want our children to be like and how we hope their lives will unfold. We often project on them how we would have liked ourselves and our lives to be different. We dream that they may overcome the pitfalls we've encountered and rise above the challenges we've faced. We want them to have the best life can offer. Our children are precious jewels we hold for a while for safekeeping and then release them into the world to behold their beauty.

In his masterful book, *The Prophet,* Kahlil Gibran writes:

Your children are not your children.

They are the sons and daughters of life's longing for itself.

You may give them your love but not your thoughts,

For they have their own thoughts.

You may house their bodies but not their souls,

For their souls dwell in the house of tomorrow, which
   you cannot visit, not even in your dreams.

You may strive to be like them but seek not to make
   them like you.

For life goes not backward nor tarries with yesterday.

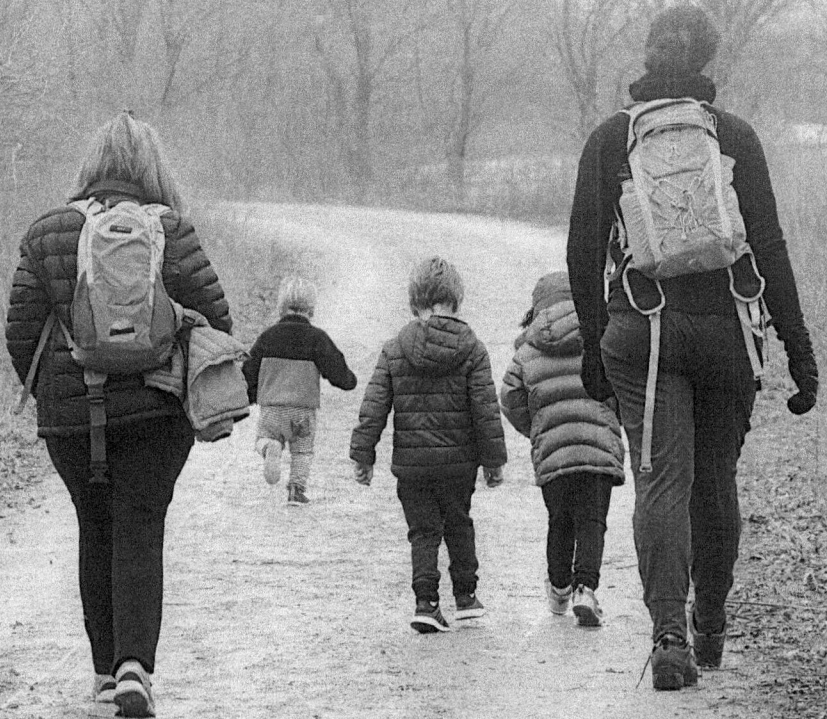

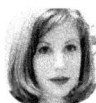

Megan's Mindful-ish Moment: Parenting and Acceptance

One of the most important, yet most difficult to process piece of parenting advice I can give you is this: your kid is not you. Childless people find it very annoying when their friends with kids say things like, "Oh, you wouldn't understand this unless you've had kids," but in this case, it's true. Before Luca was born, I thought I grasped the obvious truth that, despite that the fact that a child has grown inside of you and possesses half your genetic material, that child may differ from you in several ways. I always believed I would make a great parent because, unlike some people, I remember being a child and have a fairly comprehensive written record of my childhood, in the form of diaries, starting from the age of six. What I didn't realize was that these recollections would be helpful only if I were parenting *myself*. Almost from the moment of Luca's birth, I realized that this would not be the case.

These days, when I introduce myself to other parents as Luca's mom, they often say, "Yeah, I figured as much. She looks just like you." During her earlier years, this never happened. Although for her first few months, Luca resembled almost every other newborn baby in that eyebrow-less alien kind of way, it soon becomes abundantly clear that she was, physically, almost a carbon copy of her daddy. This is not a bad thing. I found Dave aesthetically pleasing enough to promise to look at his face every day for the rest of our lives. However, I would have liked some sort of proof that Luca is mine besides the fact I saw her come out of my vagina. The only people who told me, "She looks so much like you," were the ones who have never met Dave.

And Luca is not only like Daddy on the outside. Often, I feel he has a better sense of how her mind works than I do. Especially when she was younger, there were many times when I found myself at my wit's end, trying to teach Luca something or elicit some response, and she just didn't seem to get it. Dave would get home, and I'd tell him what I'd been struggling with. "I've said this to her in every way I can think of. Is it possible she doesn't understand what I'm saying to her?" Yes, according to Dave, it was possible. He would take a moment talking to her, and sure enough, the next moment she'd be saying, "Please, may I have some more milk?" or picking up her toys, or saying or doing whatever it was I just spent 20 minutes trying to persuade her to say or do.

I think that Dave has such a knack for knowing what's going on inside our daughter's head because she is so much like him. I often have to fight the urge to get frustrated with her when she's scared or resistant in a new situation. I feel like if I could explain enough about her new school or our upcoming vacation or her classmate's birthday party, it would alleviate her fears. When it doesn't, sometimes I feel like I'm talking to a stranger, possible one for whom English is not her first language. Dave can treat Luca with the utmost patience because he knows what it's like to feel anxious about change and awkward in social settings.

On the other hand, sometimes Luca will do something so inexplicable that neither Dave nor I can understand it. One notable example of this was her extreme and unaccountable fear of Dave's father, Don. For almost five years, whenever Don would come to our house, as soon as Luca heard his voice, she would start to scream or cry. When they were in the same room, Luca would squeeze her eyes shut as if she were trying to convince herself that if she couldn't see her grandfather, he wouldn't be there. She eventually deigned to sit at the dinner table with him, but only if the table was large enough that she didn't need to sit beside or across from him.

Dave and I had many conversations speculating about Luca's

baffling behavior. Was Don too loud and boisterous for our shy child? Did she object to the sheer quantity of his facial hair? She'd seen him at least once a month since she was born, so it's not as though he was a new character in her life. It's not as if we went into her room every night and said, "If we hear you jumping on the bed at 2 am again, Pop-Pop is going to come and throw you in a sack, and the next thing you know, you'll be in a big muddy field with big muddy dogs, dressed like the poster child for Army Surplus and shooting at ducks." No. We told her, "Pop-Pop is your family. He loves you." We'd even drawn the natural connections between Don and Santa Claus, as they are both nice bearded men who give you presents. No dice. Luca was not going to sit on the lap of either of those dudes. This was unfortunate for her, as I felt reasonably certain that Don would buy her a pony if she asked him for one.

All joking aside, it is a heartbreaking prospect to think that you may never truly understand your child, and even worse to contemplate that, someday, she may begin to agree with that assessment. I know that there are some hopes and dreams Dave and I had for Luca that we may have to let go. Since she has some trouble picking up social cues, she may never fully appreciate Dave's brand of sarcastic humor. Since she feels uneasy leaving her comfort zone, she may never want to go to the same kind of precollege sleepaway camps that were so formative to my adolescent life. It's not as though Dave and I are perfect people and want her to share all our traits. Unlike Luca, I was very attuned to social cues as a child, but along with this (and perhaps because of it), I was also ultra-sensitive and apt to take offense even when none was meant.

I liked being the center of attention, craved novelty, and could be a little scattered. Luca is a careful observer, and values routine and organization. An artistic child, I once spent months on commis-

STRESS LESS LIVE BETTER

sion to produce cat sketches for my classmates. Luca will lose interest in coloring after a few minutes, but she can read a diagram to create such complex structures with her magnetic blocks that I would have trouble duplicating them. Luca has an incredible internal compass while I couldn't find my way out of a paper bag. My way is no better or worse than her way, and I don't *need* for her to be like me. But sometimes, I feel as though I *want* her to be like me, even if it meant she shared some of my weaknesses, because then I feel I could be a better parent to her.

Letting go of the expectation that your child will be just like you is one of the kindest things you can do for him. If you don't, your child could feel like he is forever disappointing you because it will be impossible to meet your expectations. Your child may think or behave in a way that seems completely foreign to you, but that may not be a bad thing. My mom recently pointed out that if your child seems too familiar to you, you may make assumptions about what she is feeling based on your own experiences, and thus, may be completely off-base.

Six Months Later

One Sunday morning several months ago, we were planning to meet up with Dave's parents for pancakes. Luca declared, "I'm not going to be afraid of Pop-Pop anymore." And true to her word, from that moment forward, she wasn't. Now she will greet him, look straight into his eyes without anxiety, converse with him, and even hug him goodbye. Dave and I couldn't imagine what affected this transformation. Luca just changed.

And over the recent months, since I wrote the above section, Luca has changed in other ways, too. Time after time, she has shown more confidence and independence, accepting changes in her routine, initiating play with other children, and speaking to new acquaintances. She is beginning to understand sarcasm because she knows when Daddy is teasing her and when he's serious. She's even crafting her brand of humor, inventing silly jokes and songs. We thought she would be timid and unsettled starting Sunday school at a church she'd never attended before, with children and teachers she had never met. Contrary to what we expected, she sailed off without a backward glance, not even letting us walk her to her new classroom.

As parents, we believe we know our children inside and out. When they are young, we probably do know them better than anyone else does. This conviction may cause us to make judgments and predictions about our children based on past experiences with them. We need to occasionally put aside our hopes and fears, our regrets and past observations, and endeavor to "be the witness" for our children as well as ourselves. If we can get past what we think we know about our children, and see them as an outside observer would, what we notice may surprise us. The Luca I see in *this* present moment is different in some ways than the Luca from last year. In other ways, she remains the same child she has always been—inquisitive and affectionate, with music in her soul. The biggest difference is that she's beginning to let others see those personality traits her family sees every day.

Perhaps your child is trying your patience in this present moment. Maybe you feel convinced that you have the most colicky baby in history. Maybe your toddler runs away from you in the grocery store, or causes a ruckus in the restaurant, and you fear you'll never be able to take him anywhere. Remember, this, too, shall pass. That can be a bittersweet thing. At 5, Luca will still crawl in my lap and cuddle me, but I know the tween years aren't far away. Then again, when she's 8 or 9, Luca and I may be able to share things she's a bit young for at the moment, like reading Harry Potter, making friendship bracelets, or going to a Taylor Swift concert.

Six months ago, I was advising you to remember that your child is not you. I still agree with that. Appreciate your child for who she is, not for the ways she reminds you of yourself. Six months ago, I was coming to terms with letting go of some of the dreams I had for Luca. I still think that's important, but only because Luca is going to have her own dreams.

Trying to notice the present moment without judgment can fight against our impulses as parents. Moms at a group tummy time will notice how a girl baby gains the attention of the boy babies and say, "She's going to be a heartbreaker!" A toddler might measure in the 98% percentile in height at his two-year checkup, and his dad will say, "He's going to be a basketball player like his old man!" An older child might show a preference for a certain type of music or way of dressing, and his parent might worry that, someday, he'll find trouble or trouble will find him. But our children are always changing. Who knows what they will like, or be like tomorrow, next month, when they're teenagers?

Babies and young children are naturally great at living in the moment. This can sometimes be a drawback, such as when they cry like the world is ending if they don't get that cupcake *right this instant*. But it can also be an incredible benefit if we let them act as a constant reminder to be more mindful.

No doubt about it, I still have a lot left to accomplish in my life. I have dreams that can still be fulfilled. But no matter how many times I silently repeat "*Ohm Bhavam Namah*," I know that certain avenues and prospects are closed to me. Most of the time, I'm okay with that. Children, on the other hand, truly *are* fields of infinite possibility. And I can't wait to find out what possibilities my child will want to explore next.

Motherhood and Mindfulness

The more we accept ourselves, the more we can listen to and respect our children and other people in our lives for who they are, without judgment and criticism. Learning and practicing the mindfulness skills in this book can help us cope more skillfully with motherhood and other life-altering changes. Gandhi said, "Become the change you want to see in the world." May the practices and ideas in this book bring you closer to having a peaceful and joy-filled life and becoming the person and mom you want to be.

Namaste!

from Megan and Diane.

References

Borysenko, J. Z. (1995). *The power of the mind to heal*. Hay House, Inc.

Bregman, L., & Newman, S. (2015). *The mindful mom-to-be: a modern doula's guide to building a healthy foundation from pregnancy through birth*. Emmaus, PA: Rodale.

Bryant, F. B., & Veroff, J. (2017). *Savoring: A new model of positive experience*. Psychology Press.

Chopra, D., Hay, S., Newton-John, O., Frank, R., Chopra, M., & Chopra, G. (2007). *The seven spiritual laws of success*. New World Library.

Crenshaw, D. (2008). *The myth of multitasking: how doing it all gets nothing done*. San Francisco: Jossey-Bass.

Davis, M., Eshelman, E. R., & McKay, M. (2019). *The relaxation & stress reduction workbook*. Oakland, CA: New Harbinger Publications, Inc.

Domar, A. D., & Dreher, H. (1997). *Healing mind, healthy woman: Using the mind-body connection to manage stress and take control of your life*. Delta.

Dunnewold, A., & Sanford, D. (2010). *Life Will Never Be The Same: The Real Mom's Postpartum Survival Guide*. Real Moms Ink.

Dyer, W. W. (2010). *The power of intention*. Hay House, Inc.

Dyer, W. W. (2009). *Wisdom of the Ages: A Modern Master Brings Eternal Truths Into Everyday Life*. Harper Collins.

Fielding, H. (1996). *Bridget Jones's diary: a novel*. London: Picador.

Garland, E. L., Gaylord, S. A., Palsson, O., Faurot, K., Mann, J. D., & Whitehead, W. E. (2012). Therapeutic mechanisms of a mindfulness-based treatment for IBS: effects on visceral sensitivity, catastrophizing, and affective processing of pain sensations. *Journal of behavioral medicine, 35*(6), 591-602.

Greenland, S. K. (2013). *The mindful child: how to help your kid manage stress and become happier, kinder, and more compassionate*. New York: Atria Paperback.

Henry, L. (2017, October 26). The #NoMakeup Movement: Good For You, Not For Me. Retrieved from https://www.scarymommy.com/no-makeup-movement-good-for-you-not-for-me/.

Huffington, A. S. (2017). *The sleep revolution: transforming your life, one night at a time.* New York: Harmony Books.

Jennings, P. A. (2015). *Mindfulness for teachers: simple skills for peace and productivity in the classroom.* New York: W.W. Norton & Company.

Kabat-Zinn, J., & Hanh, T. N. (2009). *Full catastrophe living: Using the wisdom of your body and mind to face stress, pain, and illness.* Delta.

Kabat-Zinn, J. (2003). Mindfulness-based interventions in context: past, present, and future. *Clinical psychology: Science and practice, 10*(2), 144-156.

Kabat-Zinn, J. (1982). An outpatient program in behavioral medicine for chronic pain patients based on the practice of mindfulness meditation: Theoretical considerations and preliminary results. *General hospital psychiatry, 4*(1), 33-47.

Katz, A. (2017). *Hot mess to mindful mom: 40 ways to find balance and joy in your every day.* New York: Skyhorse Publishing.

Peterson, L. G., & Pbert, L. (1992). Effectiveness of a meditation-based stress reduction program in the treatment of anxiety disorders. *Am J Psychiatry, 149*(7), 936-43.

Northrup, C. (2012). *The wisdom of menopause.* Hay House, Inc.

Northrup, C. (2010). *Women's bodies, women's wisdom.* Hay House, Inc.

Quoidbach, J., Berry, E. V., Hansenne, M., & Mikolajczak, M. (2010). Positive emotion regulation and well-being: Comparing the impact of eight savoring and dampening strategies. *Personality and individual differences, 49*(5), 368-373.

Ruiz, D. M., & Mills, J. (2010). *The four agreements: A practical guide to personal freedom* (Vol. 1). Amber-Allen Publishing.

de Saint-Exupéry, A. (2018). *The Little Prince: A new translation by Michael Morpurgo.* Random House.

Sales, N. J. (2017). *American girls: social media and the secret lives of teenagers.* New York: Vintage Books, a division of Penguin Random House LLC.

Sanford, D. (2017). *Stress Less, Live Better: 5 Simple Steps to Ease Anxiety, Worry, and Self-Criticism.* Praeclarus Press.

Segal, Z. V., & Teasdale, J. (2018). *Mindfulness-based cognitive therapy for depression.* Guilford Publications.

Sichel, D., & Driscoll, J. W. (2000). *Women's moods, women's minds: what every woman must know about hormones, the brain, and emotional health.* Quill.

Siegel, R. D. (2009). *The mindfulness solution: Everyday practices for everyday problems.* Guilford Press.

Teasdale, J. D., Williams, J. M. G., & Segal, Z. V. (2014). *The mindful way workbook: An 8-week program to free yourself from depression and emotional distress.* Guilford Publications.

Teasdale, J. D., Segal, Z. V., Williams, J. M. G., Ridgeway, V. A., Soulsby, J. M., & Lau, M. A. (2000). Prevention of relapse/recurrence in major depression by mindfulness-based cognitive therapy. *Journal of consulting and clinical psychology, 68*(4), 615.

Tolle, E. (2004). *The power of now: A guide to spiritual enlightenment.* New World Library.

Vieten, C. (2009). *Mindful motherhood: practical tools for staying sane during pregnancy and your child's first year.* Petaluma, CA: Noetic Books, Institute of Noetic Sciences.

About the Authors

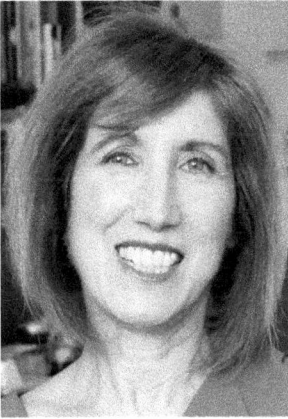

Dr. Diane Sanford is a psychologist, author, educator, and mom. An expert in perinatal mood and anxiety disorders, she learned the importance of self-care in maintaining health and wellbeing while treating pregnant and postpartum moms, but kept searching for more effective ways to reduce anxiety, worry, and self-criticism. For the past decade, she has focused on mindfulness-based solutions to remedy stress and negative thinking. Based on her experiences with hundreds of clients, training from different mindfulness and mind-body health teachers, and her own life's journey, this book offers professional guidance and personal insights that will teach you how to stress less and enjoy life more.

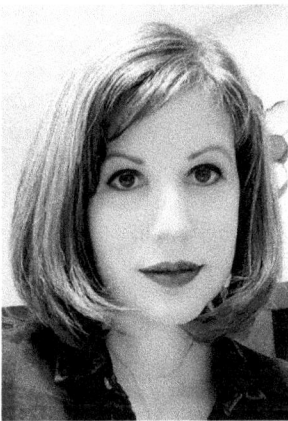

Megan Lauer Demsky is a voracious reader, foodie, shoe collector, and Shakespeare buff. She holds a B.A. in English Literature from Bard College and has worked as a writing consultant for a university. One of the first to benefit from Diane's Stress Less, Live Better program, Megan has been practicing mindfulness for over five years. She lives in the St. Louis area with her husband, daughter, and two ungrateful rescue pets.